ISBN 978-0-484-28185-0
PIBN 10683305

MARYLAND
Medical Journal

Medicine and Surgery

The Medical Journal Company
Publishers
BALTIMORE   WASHINGTON

Volume Fifty-Nine
Number Seven

JULY, 1916

Annual Subscription
Two Dollars

Obstipation Following Operation

is *psychologically* depressing to the patient and causes him to "wonder if the operation was successful." Thus, dissatisfaction with the surgeon's result often arises both with the patient and with the family doctor. The patient becomes morbid, and even a hypochondriac, and "wonders if he will ever get well."

This is in addition to the *pathology* of the condition, namely, the autotoxemia arising from the obstipation, but INTEROL, as part of the postoperative treatment, coaxes the anesthetic-deranged peristalsis back to normal, at the same time softening, and then *lubricating* the feces around bends and angulations in the gut, making possible easy bowel movement, without straining at stool.

Some of our professional friends commence the INTEROL treatment one to three days following operation, and continue its use after the patient leaves the hospital.* Eventually, it is diminished and finally discontinued,—INTEROL, in most cases, does not have to be taken forever.

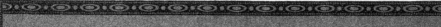
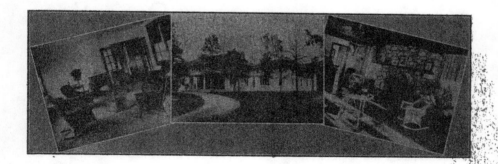

MARYLAND MEDICAL JOURNAL

FOR JULY, 1916

VOL. LIX   *Entered at the Baltimore Postoffice as Second-Class Matter*   No. 7

CONTENTS

Terms: $2.00 a Year   THE MEDICAL JOURNAL CO.
Professional Building   Baltimore, Md.   Index to Ads. Page ii

INDEX TO ADVERTISERS

When writing, say you saw advertisement in the MARYLAND MEDICAL JOURNAL.

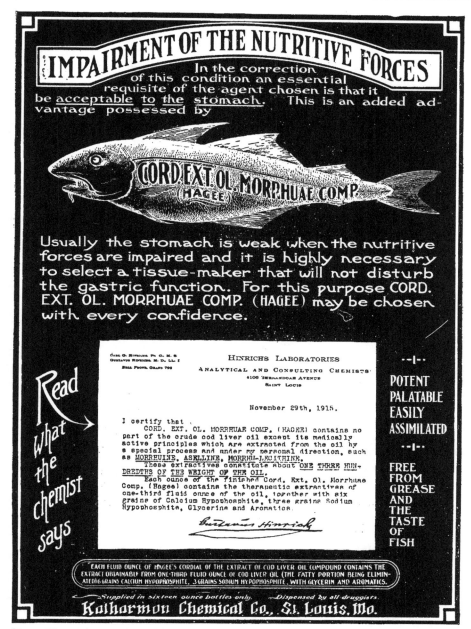
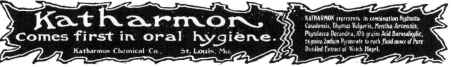

Medical Society Meetings

MARYLAND

NOTE.—Secretaries are requested to advise us promptly of the election of new officers in their respective Societies, that due announcement may be made in the JOURNAL.

Except where otherwise stated, the Medical Societies of Baltimore meet at the Medical and Chirurgical Faculty building, 1211 Cathedral Street.

MEDICAL AND CHIRURGICAL FACULTY OF MARYLAND. President, J. WHITRIDGE WILLIAMS, M.D.; Secretary, JOSEPH I. FRANCE, M.D.

Baltimore City Medical Society

President, CHAS. E. SADTLER, M.D.; Vice-President, F. H. BAETJER, M.D.; Secretary, EMIL NOVÁK, M.D.; Treasurer, W. S. GARDNER, M.D.; Censors, C. E. BRACK, M.D., O. B. PANCOAST, M.D., R. WINSLOW, M.D.; Delegates, GORDON WILSON, M.D., C. F. BURNHAM, M.D., J. M. H. ROWLAND, M.D., JOHN T. KING, M.D., W. A. FISHER, JR., M.D., R. FAYERWEATHER, M.D., H. FRIEDENWALD, M.D., J. H. PLEASANTS, M.D., S. McCLEARY, M.D., J. STAIGE DAVIS, M.D., W. E. BRINTON, M.D.

SECTION OF CLINICAL MEDICINE AND SURGERY. 1st and 3d Fridays, 8.30 P. M.; October to May. Chairman, J. STAIGE DAVIS, M.D.; Secretary, E. B. FREEMAN, M.D.

SECTION OF DERMATOLOGY. 3d Wednesdays. Chairman, J. WILIAMS LORD, M.D.; Secretary, L. R. PELS, M.D.

SECTION OF GYNECOLOGY AND OBSTETRICS. 2d Fridays in October, December, February and April. Chairman, J. M. H. ROWLAND, M.D.; Secretary, EMIL NOVÁK, M.D.

SECTION OF LARYNGOLOGY. 4th Fridays monthly, 8.30 o'clock. Chairman, LEE COHEN, M.D.; Secretary, G. W. MITCHELL, M.D.

SECTION OF MEDICAL EXAMINERS. 3d Fridays in November and March. Chairman, J. D. IGLEHART, M.D.; Secretary, W. E. MAGRUDER, M.D.

SECTION OF NEUROLOGY. 2d Friday, monthly. Chairman, C. M. BYRNES, M.D.; Secretary, D. V. STUART, M.D.

SECTION OF OPHTHALMOLOGY AND OTOLOGY. 3d Wednesdays. Chairman, J. W. DOWNEY, JR., M.D.; Secretary, L. B. WHITHAM, M.D.

County Societies

ALLEGANY COUNTY MEDICAL SOCIETY. President, J. T. JOHNSON, M.D., Cumberland: Secretary-Treasurer, M. J. SIMMONS, M.D., Cumberland, Md.; Delegate, A. LEO FRANKLIN, M.D.

ANNE ARUNDEL COUNTY MEDICAL SOCIETY. President, T. H. BRAYSHAW, M.D., Glenburnie, Md.; Secretary, L. B. HENKEL, JR., M.D., Annapolis, Md.; Treasurer, F. H. THOMPSON, M.D., Annapolis, Md.; Delegate, C. R. WINTERSON, M.D.

BALTIMORE COUNTY MEDICAL SOCIETY. President, G. C. McCORMICK, M.D., Sparrows Point, Md.; Secretary, J. C. MONMONIER, M.D., Catonsville, Md.; Treasurer, F. C. ELDRED, M.D., Sparrows Point, Md.; Delegate, H. L. NAYLOR, M.D., Towson, Md.

CALVERT COUNTY MEDICAL SOCIETY. President, COMPTON WILSON, M.D., Friendship, Md.; Secretary-Treasurer, J. W. LEITCH, M.D., Huntingtown, Md.; Delegate, P. BRISCOE, M.D.

CAROLINE COUNTY MEDICAL SOCIETY. President, W. W. GOLDSBOROUGH, M.D., Greensboro, Md.; Secretary-Treasurer, J. R. DOWNES, M.D., Preston, Md.; Delegate, H. W. B. ROWE, M.D., Hillsboro, Md.

CARROLL COUNTY MEDICAL SOCIETY. President, C. R. FOUTZ, M.D., Westminster, Md.; Secretary-Treasurer, H. M. FITZHUGH, M.D., Westminster, Md.; Delegate, M. D. NORRIS, M.D.

CECIL COUNTY MEDICAL SOCIETY. President, A. H. CANTWELL, M.D., North East, Md.: Secretary-Treasurer. H. BRATTON, M.D., Elkton, Md.; Delegate, G. H. RICHARDS, M.D.

CHARLES COUNTY MEDICAL SOCIETY. President, JOHN W. MITCHELL, M.D., Pomonkey, Md.; Secretary-Treasurer, THOMAS S. OWEN, M.D., La Plata, Md.; Delegate, L. C. CARRICO, M.D.

DORCHESTER COUNTY MEDICAL SOCIETY. President, GUY STEELE, M.D., Cambridge, Md.; Secretary-Treasurer, W. H. HOUSTON, M.D., Fishing Creek, Md.; Delegate, E. E. WOLFF, M.D., Cambridge, Md.

FREDERICK COUNTY MEDICAL SOCIETY. President, M. A. BIRELY, M.D., Thurmont, Md.; Secretary, B. O. THOMAS, M.D., Frederick, Md.; Treasurer, W. C. JOHNSON, M.D., Frederick, Md.; Delegate, J. C. ROUTSON, M.D. January, April, August and November.

HARFORD COUNTY MEDICAL SOCIETY. President, A. F. VAN BIBBER, M.D., Belair, Md.; Secretary-Treasurer, CHARLES BAGLEY, M.D., Bagley, Md.; Delegate, W. S. ARCHER, M.D. 2d Wednesdays in January, March, May, July, September and November.

HOWARD COUNTY MEDICAL SOCIETY. President, W. C. STONE, M.D., Ellicott City, Md.; Secretary-Treasurer, W. L. CISSEL, M.D., Highland, Md.; Delegate, W. R. WHITE. Meetings quarterly first Tuesdays in January, April, July and October.

KENT COUNTY MEDICAL SOCIETY. President, H. G. SIMPERS, M.D., Chestertown, Md.; Secretary-Treasurer, F. B. HINES, M.D., Chestertown, Md.; Delegate, F. B. HINES, M.D.

MONTGOMERY COUNTY MEDICAL SOCIETY. President, F. N. HENDERSON, M.D., Rockville, Md.; Secretary-Treasurer, C. H. MANNAR, M.D., Rockville, Md.; Delegate, W. L. LEWIS, M.D. 3d Tuesdays in April and October.

PRINCE GEORGE'S COUNTY MEDICAL SOCIETY. President, H. B. McDONNELL, M.D., College Park, Md.; Secretary, S. M. McMILLAN, M.D., Riverdale, Md.; Treasurer, W. ALLEN GRIFFITH, M.D., Berwyn, Md.; Delegate, L. A. GRIFFITH, M.D. 2d Saturday of every second month.

QUEEN ANNE'S COUNTY MEDICAL SOCIETY. President, C. P. KEMP, M.D., Stevensville, Md.; Secretary-Treasurer, H. F. McPHERSON, M.D., Centerville, Md.; Delegate, J. W. STACK, M.D.

SOMERSET COUNTY MEDICAL SOCIETY. President, R. R. NORRIS, M.D., Crisfield, Md.; Secretary-Treasurer, H. M. LANKFORD, M.D., Princess Anne, Md.; Delegate, C. W. WAINWRIGHT, M.D. 1st Tuesday in October, at Princess Anne.

TALBOT COUNTY MEDICAL SOCIETY. President, SAMUEL TRIPPE, M.D., Royal Oak, Md.; Secretary-Treasurer, A. McC. STEVENS, M.D., Easton, Md.; Delegate, J. A. STEVENS, M.D. Annual meeting 3d Tuesday in November and semi-annual meeting 3d Tuesday in May.

WASHINGTON COUNTY MEDICAL SOCIETY. President. W. B. MORRISON, M.D., Hagerstown, Md.; Secretary, V. D. MILLER, M.D., Hagerstown, Md.; Treasurer, W. B. MORRISON, M.D., Hagerstown, Md.; Delegate, V. D. MILLER, M.D. 2d Thursdays of February, May, September and November.

WICOMICO COUNTY MEDICAL SOCIETY. President. J. M. ELDERDICE, M.D., Mardela Springs; Secretary and Treasurer, H. S. WAILES, M.D., Salisbury, Md.; Delegate, G. W. TODD, M.D.

WORCESTER COUNTY MEDICAL SOCIETY. President, R. LEE HALL, M.D., Pocomoke City, Md.; Secretary and Treasurer, E. E. WISEHART, M.D., Snow Hill, Md.; Delegate, J. L. RILEY, M.D., Snow Hill, Md.

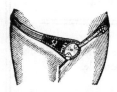
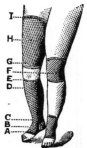
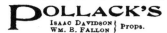

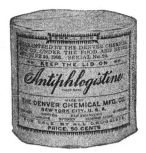
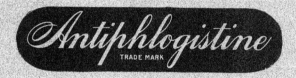

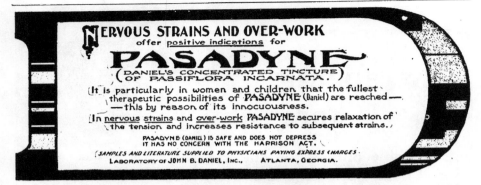

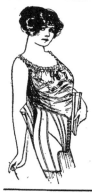
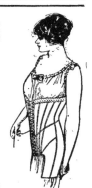

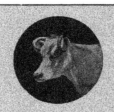
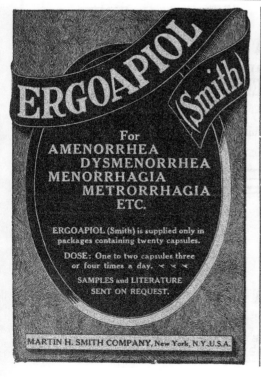
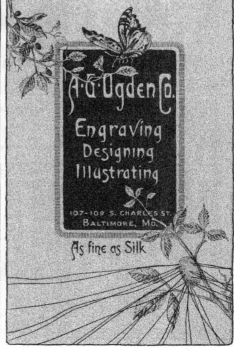

MARYLAND
MEDICAL JOURNAL
A Journal of Medicine and Surgery

| Vol. LIX, No. 7 | BALTIMORE, JULY, 1916 | Whole No. 1178 |

THE EVOLUTION OF NURSING.*

By Harvey G. Beck, M.D.

WHEN Sister Imelda invited me to deliver an address on this occasion I assured her of my high appreciation of the honor. My pleading that I should find an excuse to be out of the city on the day of the commencement was without avail. With her usual tack and diplomacy she simply remarked "Think it over." Now, I should like to know who, after solemn, serious thought, could refrain from accepting an opportunity to pay a tribute to the noble cause these worthy, self-sacrificing women of the Sisters of Mercy espouse, and to add a few words of praise and commendation to the young ladies who so studiously and diligently pursued their course of instruction at the Training School of the Mercy Hospital for three long years, and whose graduation we are here to honor today.

In glancing over the literature to find some basis for my remarks I was imbued with the fact that the history of nursing is one of the most interesting subjects I have ever delved into. Nursing for thousands of years has been so closely interwoven with science and religion, war and pestilence, ignorance and superstition, and is so replete with notable characters of men and women whose acts of heroism, self-sacrificing love and devotion to the care of suffering humanity, that it makes this field for study extremely broad in domain and rich in material. Indeed, it was with fear and trepidation that I chose for my subject "The Evolution of Nursing," feeling that I might not be able to keep my remarks within that soul-saving time limit Professor Hadley recently referred to.

One day a visiting clergyman who was to preach before the students at Yale University asked how long he was expected to talk. "Of course, we put no time limit upon you," replied President Hadley, "but we have a feeling here at Yale that no souls are saved after the first twenty minutes."

---

*Address delivered at the Commencement of the Mercy Hospital Training School for Nurses, May 25, 1915.

Should I fail to save every soul here from going to sleep, you will have to blame it on my ardor and enthusiasm over the subject.

Nursing as an art is said to be the oldest occupation for women; as a science, the youngest branch of the medical profession. The first mother performed for her little ones all those services that made it possible for them to live, and to these maternal cares may be attributed the foundation from which the profession of nursing has developed.

According to John Fiske, the longer period of time during which the human infant is helpless and dependent evokes a prolonged and enduring tenderness in the parents, with the resultant superior development of character. In addition to this parental instinct, there is a second—that of mutual aid, which is found in animals as well as in man, and tends to the preservation of species. This latter has even been observed among savage races. In the animal kingdom one may see splendid examples of "first aid" to the injured. Apes stop bleeding by compression; birds have been known to treat fracture of the leg by splints and grasses, and injured deer travel many miles to immerse an inflamed wound in water. A forrester who observed this latter fact was responsible for the beginning of the water cure in Europe. Cats and dogs when not well eat familiar grasses and weeds. It may thus be observed that animals, through instinct, possess a vast fund of practical knowledge. The same was true of primitive man until the instinct was crowded out by over-civilization. In the remote mountain districts at the present day there still exists a type of mother and grandmother who, with their intimate knowledge of healing herbs, serve as both doctor and nurse for their families. As the knowledge of herbs became more extended, there were those who devoted their time to healing, such as the medicine man, witches and sorcerers, priests and priestesses of pagan nations. These had associated with them assistants, usually the women of the tribe, who were skilful in the dressing of wounds, and acted somewhat in the capacity of nurse. Among these practitioners there were those who were good and evilly disposed, and their art became known, respectively, as "black" or "white" magic, a distinction which lasted throughout the Middle Ages.

Among savage tribes practical nursing of a certain kind was not to be despised. They could dress wounds, massage the various parts of the body, make helpful teas from herbs, and even give sweat baths. Bleeding and cupping, amputation of limbs, trephining and many other operations that, in the present day are considered grave, were successfully performed. Vaccination against smallpox has been practiced from time immemorial by certain savage tribes.

From earliest times to the Christian era very little is definitely known about the special duties of the nurse; yet there is a reference in the writings of a physician of India, Charaka, 320 B. C., who mentions a nurse as one of the four requisites for a cure and defines her four qualifications—"knowledge of the manner in which drugs are prepared, cleverness, devotedness to the patient and purity of mind and body"—qualities as essential today as they were in the days of Charaka.

During the pre-Christian era the historical records of nursing are broken and incomplete, but beginning with the early Christian workers there is a continuity of record up to the present day, a period of nearly two thousand years.

During the early Christian era the work of nursing was divided quite evenly between men and women. Among the first church orders of women engaged in nursing were the Deaconesses, Widows and Nuns. Later among the men were the military and religious orders, who devoted much time to nursing through medieval times.

Phebe, the first deaconess, of whom St. Paul said, "She hath been a succourer of many and of myself also," was one of the distinguished personages of her day. Besides performing many secular and clerical duties, it is said of her that she was the first parish worker, friendly visitor and district nurse, and from her day the work of visiting nursing has been in continuous practice.

The origin of hospitals may be traced back to the order of deaconesses, who not only visited the sick, but also brought them into their own homes to be cared for. The modern hospital grew out of this system, first, by using rooms in private houses. then additions or cloisters added to the homes, and finally separate hospital buildings. The necessity for both hospitals and nursing was occasioned by the pestilences, pilgrimages and crusades.

Pestilences and pilgrimages were closely associated, since the latter was the great source of spreading epidemics. Certain of the religious orders devoted themselves to nursing of the sick and maimed on their pilgrimages. This led to the establishment of hospices and hospitals. Among the patrican nurses were two distinguished women—Fabiola, who built a hospital in Rome, and Paula, who built hospitals for the pilgrims, one on the road to Bethlehem and one in Jerusalem, and who herself looked after the sick.

One of the earliest known instances of nursing in the noble struggle against misery waged by the early Christians was during a violent pestilence in Alexandria between the years 249 and 263 A. D.

A century later, during a frightful epidemic of the plague, St. Ephrem bought, from money donated, 300 beds, which he placed in public porticos and galleries, thus establishing the first hospital in the strict sense as the term is used today. At about this same period, on account of the numerous lepers and a great famine, Basil established the most notable hospital of all the early institutions. The staff consisted of nurses, doctors, carriers and artisans.

Beginning with the fifth century, or the rise of monasticism, there is a wonderful record of religious nursing of a thousand years and more. This extended through the Middle Ages, with their vast, wealthy and beautiful monasteries and hospitals and the supremacy of monastic orders, and down to the present day, when, on account of the modern sciences, new economic and social adjustments, this system of nursing no longer obtains. However, these old religious orders are still models of organizations and discipline.

Medicine as well as nursing was almost entirely within the province of the church, and both were conducted on a high plane until the latter part of the seventeenth century, when the status and competence of the female attendant had sunk as low as the hospital in which they served. This was almost universally the case outside of the Roman Catholic orders, in which discipline and decency still prevailed.

The period between the latter part of the seventeenth century and the middle of the nineteenth century was known as the "dark age" of sick nursing. A brief description of conditions as they prevailed in several of the world's oldest and most famous hospitals will best serve to illustrate the chaos and downfall of both medicine and nursing during this age.

Hotel Dieu, a leading hospital in Paris, was established in 650 A. D., and for twelve centuries the Augustinian Sisters served the institution. Their lives were so intimately intertwined with their work that they had no other home, for here they lived from the day of their profession to the day of their death. Their lot was needlessly hard, without professional instruction, intellectual life or outside amusement. A little over one hundred years ago the servant nurse was introduced. The condition of the hospital at this time was in an appalling state. Tenon describes it as containing 1219 beds, 733 of which were large, holding from two to six patients, and 486 smaller ones. They stood in two, three or four rows, the small and large being mixed together, and so unevenly placed that some could only be reached from the foot. others from the side. In 1873 a famous Vienna surgeon in describing his rounds said that in one bed he had noticed one patient dead, two others dying and one convalescent. The beds were of wood, with shelves at head and foot to hold patient's medicines, and made with heavy straw mattresses and a feather bed on top. White muslin bed curtains were used in summer and red serge in winter. The huge beds occupied so much space that cleaning was impossible. The walls were filthy with the expectoration of the patients, and it was impossible to prevent bed bugs. Itch and scabies were general. The former was of such a malign character that it caused suppuration and gangrene and destroyed many eyes. The operating-room. where they trephine, cut and amputate, contains at once those who have been and are to be operated upon as well as those undergoing operations. They all see the preparations for torture and hear the cries of agony—all this before the days of anesthesia. The secular nurse had poor and inadequate rooms, and when sick was placed in the loathsome ward beds with the

patients.   The historian refers to other wretched conditions in
the hospital which he says are indescribable.

In England conditions were no better.   Indeed, there was practically an absence of nursing after the suppression of the convents
and the expulsion of the religious sisters from the hospitals during
the reign of Henry VIII in 1523.   In 1665, 65,000 died of the
plague in England.   Smallpox also regularly caused ten per cent.
of all deaths.

For seven hundred years famine and pestilence were horribly
associated.   The houses, damp and cold, without ventilation or
drainage, invited illness, but in time of pestilence stricken persons
were locked in them to die or recover without nursing or medical
aid.   The pesthouse, which, fortunately, is now passing out of
existence in civilized countries, was a place of untold horrors.

Ignorance of disease and superstition in medicine reigned
supreme at this period.   Going back through ages the healing god
had given place to the healing saint, and now the saint was sometimes displaced by the King.   For a long time the "King's Touch"
of Charles II was supposed to cure the King's evil or scrofula.
About 92,000 persons, including a man of no less intellectual
attainment than Samuel Johnson, sought his magic touch.

Hospitals were likened unto prisons, and with municipal and State
control the religious order gave way to the servant nurse.   These
were poorly housed, ill-fed, overworked and underpaid, ignorant,
untaught and unorganized, and were kept in a state of abject
degradation.   Their hours on duty were from twelve to forty-
eight, twenty-four being quite the ordinary.   The result was that
only women of the Sairey Gamp type as portrayed by Dickens
were available.

As to the duties of the nurse, let me quote some of the rules
that were enforced in St. Thomas Hospital, the institution in
which Florence Nightingale began her wonderful reform: "She
is to make all the beds on one side of the ward, and to scour and
make clean the bed and floors of the whole ward, with the tables
and forms, the passage and stairs and garrets; to assist her, she
may take such patients as the sisters shall think fit and able to
help her.   She must keep clean, scour the cans for beer, the broth
pails, pans, platters and plates, etc., fouled at dinner.   She must
attend the butler at the ringing of the beer-bell, and take with her
such patients as are able to carry the beer in safety to the ward,
and not suffer such patients to waste or embezzle it by the way,
but see that the cans be carried full into the ward; and in like
manner, at his ringing the bread-bell, she must attend and take
the just number of loaves for the patients who are entitled to it;
and also at the ringing of the cook's bell she must attend her and
receive from her the exact quantity of provisions that are appointed for each patient."

Such a regime held out quite an inducement to ward patients,
but the nurse had her emoluments as well.   At St. Thomas her
salary consisted of nine shillings seven pence a week, and beer.
At St. George's Hospital they received six pounds of bread a week,

one-half pint of milk and two pints of beer daily, and one shilling a day to buy additional food.

In Austria the same inhuman conditions existed, and still exist, in the world's renowned hospital in Vienna—the Algemeines Kraunkenhaus. There one finds the same nursing personnel. Not many years ago, while I was pursuing studies in the wards of this hospital, the nurses were highly inferior intellectually, slovenly in their habits and dress, and of the servant type. They slept in small cubicles in the wards of both male and female patients, and their meals, which they had to bring up themselves, they ate in the wards. This institution gave twenty-four hours duty, alternating with a day of three short periods.

These few glimpses into the dark period of nursing will arouse one to a fuller sense of appreciation of the remarkable evolution which has taken place in nursing in the past five or six decades. Out of chaos and degradation has emerged in this short time one of the loftiest and noblest of professions.

The establishment of a school for the special training of deaconess nurses by Pastor Fleidner and his wife, Frederike, at Kaiserwerth in 1836 marked the beginning of a new epoch. This institution soon became celebrated, and its influence was rapidly spread by Elizabeth Fry, who was so inspired with the work of Fleidner that she established a religious school for training nurses in England, and by the immortal Florence Nightingale, a pupil at Kaiserwerth, who has made nursing the model institution which it is in English-speaking countries today. Florence Nightingale, who had gone to the Crimea with thirty-four nurses, ten of whom were Sisters of Mercy, to care for the wounded on the battlefields, called attention to the inestimable value of organized and systematized nursing, and at the close of the war a fund of $250,000 was raised with which in 1860 she established a school for the education of women as nurses at St. Thomas Hospital.

In 1887 Queen Victoria gave $350,000, the surplus of the Women's Jubilee Offering, to the founding of a similar institution. The so-called Nightingale nurses soon filled vacancies in other large hospitals, and thus brought about a regeneration of English nursing.

The American schools of nursing were modeled after the English. As early as 1798 lectures were given to the nurse attendants in the New York Hospital by Dr. Valentine Seaman, but regular training schools were not established until 1873. That year one was established at Bellevue Hospital, one at New Haven and one at the Massachusetts General Hospital.

The establishment of these schools was the beginning of a new era of nursing in America. The progress from this day was in leaps and bounds. Schools were organized in rapid succession, so that at present there are at least five hundred in the United States. The course of training was conducted on a strictly ethical and scientific basis—in short, a new profession was born, unique and distinctive in character, a department of modern medical science. Today the profession of nursing in America ranks foremost in the world, and the American nurse has become the ideal. To even mention her remarkable achievement and her widespread and elevating influence in the public, domestic and social .life of our country would at once break my "soul-saving" pledge. For this information I refer you to those interesting volumes on the "History of Nursing," by two eminent American nurses, Miss Nutting and Miss Dock, and shall now proceed to what concerns us more personally on this occasion and tell you who is who today, and why.

Need I tell you who is who today? These ladies of the graduating class, their friends and sweethearts, can answer this question. Reasoning from cause to effect, I must first answer the question "why." The Sisters of Mercy are too modest to do this. Nevertheless, they are responsible for who is who today.

The order of the Sisters of Mercy was founded by Mother Catherine McAuley in Dublin in 1827. The order was first introduced in the United States in 1843.

The visitation of the sick is one of the duties of the Order of Mercy. When this order was founded, hospitals and homes for the needy were not provided as they are now, and consequently there was a necessity for somebody to look after the poor sick in their homes, and this duty Mother McAuley assigned to her daughters.

All who know the Sisters of Mercy remember the little brown visitation basket which was always seen in their hands on their visitations to the sick. Refreshments were taken and relief was rendered in whatever way it was most needed.

As already mentioned, at the outbreak of the Crimean War in 1854, Florence Nightingale asked for ten Sisters to accompany her to the Crimea. A temporary hospital was erected at Balaklava, and the Sisters nursed until the close of the war, when they were recalled to Ireland. Two Sisters died during that time, and were buried on the Crimean peninsula.

During the Spanish-American War, in 1898, twelve Sisters of Mercy entered Chickamauga Park amid 80,000 troops. These were the first women to take up nursing in that park. They were sent to the scene of war by the United States Government. Later on they were complimented by President McKinley for their efficient nursing, great kindness to the soldiers and self-sacrificing work. The order lost one of the members of the nursing corps, who was taken down with the fever and died.

They founded the old Mercy Hospital in 1871. In 1897 they opened the Nurses' Training School. Prior to that date the Sisters had done all the nursing themselves. Because of their moral and religious, in addition to their intellectual and nursing, training they are pre-eminently qualified for conducting a school for the training of nurses. It is their firm conviction that the heart as well as the head and hands must be trained, for a nurse without a heart or soul that adapts itself to this noble work is utterly unfitted for the proper exercises of her duties.

And now, to the ladies of the graudating class—well, I hardly know what to say, especially since some of them requested me to say "the real nice things about the nurses," such as Dr. Harry Friedenwald said in his address a year ago. Indeed, I should quote his address in full had he not said so much and paid so many glowing tributes. However, on second thought, I find his remarks do not apply at all to this class. For, while he was addressing the best class of nurses ever graduated up to a year ago, I am addressing a better one today, for in the very nature of the rapid evolution of nursing each succeeding class must needs be better. Therefore, let me congratulate you upon the proud distinction you have won. You have chosen a noble calling, a self-sacrificing one, altruistic in character and full of service to suffering humanity. Remember, this is only the beginning of your career. The responsibilities will now be shifted from the Sisters of Mercy to your shoulders. Bravery, courage and conviction must characterize your efforts. Practice the precepts taught by the Sisters and never allow your heart and soul to get out of the work and dampen your ardour and love of devotion to duty. You may have to sail many troubled seas, and it may be said of you, as a little girl said of me one day when a neighbor asked her how her sister Helen was. She replied, "Oh, she is well. She got well as soon as the doctor quit coming." However, you can rest assured that good, honest service is always rewarded.

Work is the keynote to success, but let me emphasize that recreation is necessary for efficient work and must not be neglected. According to Cabot, men live by work, play, love and worship. They are as essential to your individual welfare and happiness as food and raiment. Keep these requisites always in mind, and success will crown your efforts.

There is another phase of this important subject upon which I do not have time to dwell. It is the gratitude of the patients to whom your knowledge and skill is applied.

To conclude my remarks I will quote a few lines from an ode to the nurses, written by a patient of Mercy Hospital whose heart was touched with the loving and tender care she received at the hands of these nurses who are graduating today.

"Her very presence seems to help us,
  As our fevered pulse she feels,
Her soft white hand with gentle touch
  Soothes and helps our wounds to heal,
  The gentle little nurse at Mercy.

"With a heart that is true and tender,
  Her sympathies are with us in pain;
She ministers to us in suffering,
  And sends us home well again,
  The kind little nurse at Mercy.

"Blessings upon her, yes, every one,
  Is my prayer to the Father above,
Giving their lives in service to others,
  These ministering angels of love,
  The God-given nurses at Mercy."

AN ANSWER TO THE QUERY: SHALL THE CITY OF BALTIMORE SURRENDER QUARANTINE TO THE FEDERAL GOVERNMENT? *

By J. A. Nydegger,

Surgeon, United States Public Health Service.

Mr. President, and Members of the Medico-Chirurgical Faculty:

It gives me great pleasure to appear before you for the purpose of saying something on the much-discussed question, "Shall the City of Baltimore Surrender Its Quarantine to the Federal Government?" Those of you present who happen to reside in this city know this is a question to which I have paid considerable attention during the past three years.

Maritime quarantine protects more than a city; it protects an entire State, and even other States which are liable to become infected by dangerous contagious diseases by reason of persons coming from foreign places where these diseases prevail and passing through quarantine into the city or going to parts in the State outside of the city or to places in other States.

It is for this reason, gentlemen, that I put myself in the somewhat embarrassing position of writing to your president and suggesting to him to have this question placed on the program for the meeting.

I shall be as brief as possible in my remarks, and will endeavor to touch only on the most vital points of this question.

The history of quarantine is a long one, and, as originally applied, it meant 40 days detention of vessels and persons in quarantine, and comes from the Latin word "quarante," meaning forty.

To the city of Venice must be given the credit of having established the first quarantine of the world, when it put into use a quarantine against epidemic diseases coming from the East along the lines of maritime commerce in the middle of the fourteenth century. The physicians of those days knew nothing of the period of incubation of communicable diseases, and to make sure of taking no risks, all persons found suffering from any of the dangerous epidemic diseases were subjected to a like period of quarantine, namely, 40 days.

Almost from the time since quarantine was first put into effect a tendency existed to make it uniform not only in a city or country, but throughout all of the leading countries of the world. There were important commercial reasons for this as well as others, for health, quarantine and commerce have always been intimately connected. So important were these features to the welfare and prosperity of any country that France, under Louis

---

*Address delivered at the annual meeting of the Maryland Medico-Chirurgical Faculty, held in Baltimore, April 25-26, 1916.

XIV in the seventeenth century, first promulgated the order that took from its many cities and local boards of health, which maintained each a different set of quarantine rules and regulations, and gave the first general sanitary regulations for the whole of France and thus established the fact that maritime quarantine is a function to be executed by the country at large, and not by a province or city.

A step forward in the application of quarantine throughout Europe was when the first International Sanitary Conference was held in Paris in 1851, attended by the representatives of the 12 leading European countries most actively engaged in maritime commerce. This conference resulted in the formulation of a code of more scientific quarantine measures, to be enforced uniformly at the ports of all countries represented.

In 1903, at a similar congress held in Paris, 20 leading powers, including the United States, signed what is known as the International Sanitary Agreement, which provided for uniformity in the quarantine rules and administration of them in the seaports of the countries there represented. In the 19 other countries represented at this congress the matter of maritime quarantine had long since been recognized as being pre-eminently a function of the general government, and control of their quarantines has centuries ago been transferred from province and municipality to their respective governments.

The development of maritime quarantine in the United States is practically a duplicate of the development of quarantine in European and other trans-oceanic countries.

In colonial times the different Legislatures had control over the quarantines. a power which was inherited by the States and municipalities. and is still exercised by them in the ports of New York and Baltimore.

After the first sanitary conference, held in Paris in 1851, it became evident that the non-uniformity of the laws regulating quarantine in the different States of this country not only caused inconvenience to freight and passenger traffic, but was a positive menace to public safety. Some ports, for the purpose of attracting commerce, would be lax in following the strict regulations which they had imposed on themselves, while others would make mild regulations with the same object of getting trade, thus frequently admitting dangerous epidemic diseases.

In the meantime, although there were no acts passed which gave the Federal Government direct power over the quarantine at all ports of the country, the trend of all the legislation in this connection was toward this goal. A number of national quarantine acts were passed from 1799 to 1893. From time to time also acts were passed increasing the powers and broadening the shpere of work of the Federal public health service. All these acts, however, provided that the measures were for the purpose of aiding the State and municipal authorities, and did not give the Federal Government the power of supervision over them.

This was first done by the act of 1893, which gave the Secretary of the Treasury, through the Public Health Service, the power to promulgate uniform quarantine regulations for all the ports of the United States, which rules must be enforced by State and municipal authorities if they chose to undertake to enforce them, and in case of their refusal or failure to carry out these regulations, the President is empowered to detail Federal public health officers for that purpose.

This act also gave the Public Health Service the power to examine the quarantine stations of a State or municipality and their regulations. The act further forbids any decrease in the application in quarantine of the Federal regulations, but does not prevent additional requirements that may be imposed by State or municipal quarantine authorities. Also, where a State or municipality shall transfer to the United States their quarantine stations, they shall reasonably be reimbursed therefor.

Following in the footsteps of what all other maritime countries of the world a long time ago effected, the process of transferring from State and municipal to Federal control all of the quarantine stations in the United States has been steadily going on since the passage of the act of 1893. Of the grand total in the United States of 50 such stations, 48 have been transferred already, leaving but 2—New York, which is about to establish by law what it has already established in practice, and Baltimore, which stands in a class alone as being the very last city in the world to take steps to transfer its quarantine to Government control.

The city of Baltimore has been playing in great luck since 1892. At that time cholera prevailed extensively in certain European countries, and there was great danger of its introduction into the United States in the person of immigrants arriving at our ports from the places where the disease prevailed. At that time the Federal Government, recognizing the unprepared condition of this city's quarantine station and the danger of cholera gaining access to the country through it, established at Old Point Comfort, Va., a quarantine station, and came to the relief of the city, and thereby averted a threatened invasion, much to the relief of the people of Baltimore and the country at large.

Owing to the long continued state of war in several of the European countries, which in normal times furnish 90 per cent. of the immigrants arriving in the United States, and owing to the great spread of the dangerous diseases, such as typhus fever, plague, cholera and smallpox in these countries, and the great danger of these diseases being introduced into the United States in arriving immigrants, it seems imperative that some action should at once be taken by the people of Baltimore to prevent the introduction of these diseases into the city through a quarantine station, which in its present absolutely inadequate size and condition to care for any number of detained immigrants or others in case of sickness is a matter of record.

The present accommodations and inadequate equipment of the

station provides for the detention of less than 70 persons, while it not infrequently happens that from 1200 to 1500, and even 1800 immigrants, in addition to the large crews, arrive at this port on one vessel.

The question involved at present is not one of money, but health protection better than the city now has. As previously stated, this city has been playing in great luck since 1892. No dangerous diseases have been brought to the city in the meantime. If a vessel should arrive at the present time with a paltry 200 passengers, and with dangerous diseases such as have been mentioned existing among them, the quarantine station could not possibly care for this small number, and would be utterly helpless. What would be the case if a vessel should arrive with 1500 passengers under similar conditions and these people had to be detained at quarantine? What would be the result? The station would be utterly inadequate to meet the demands and afford the health protection which the people of this city and of this State and of other States are entitled to and should expect. The medical men of this State and the people should know these facts. Should I know these facts and not make them known to you, I would consider myself no longer a loyal citizen and a public health officer. I tell you there is great danger of these dangerous diseases being brought into the United States after the present European War is over.

In order to forestall the possible introduction of dangerous diseases through this port, the Government two months ago submitted to the city and the shipping interests of this city a most advantageous proportion—(1) that it would take care of Baltimore's (City) smallpox cases and all other maritime quarantinable diseases that may occur in the city at the nominal charge of $1 per day; (2) that it would purchase the quarantine station and all property belonging to it at a liberal price; (3) that it would rebuild, greatly enlarge and equip properly to care for the largest number of immigrants that may arrive on any vessel with possible dangerous diseases among them, and would increase its facilities for the disinfection and prompt dispatch of vessels, and (4) that it will continue in the service the present employes at the station, and in order to better expedite shipping, it will establish a night medical inspection service, to be in force from sundown to midnight.

The city has favorably considered the unprecedented offer on the part of the Government, submitted solely for the purpose of acquiring prompt control of the quarantine, with the view of immediately taking steps to equip it in every way and make it a modern station, fit for the protection of the health of the city of Baltimore and the country.

Should the people of this city and this State permit of this serious jeopardizing of the health of the community longer?

Should they permit the desire of possible gain to be supreme to the matter of the health of the people?

The foreign shipping interests of the port are striving to delay the actual transfer of the quarantine station to Federal control until some future date for no good or sufficient reason, claiming that the commerce of this port would be injured as compared to New York should the transfer be affected before the New York quarantine station is transferred.

The Governor of New York some months ago requested the loan by the Public Health Service of an experienced quarantine officer to take charge of the New York quarantine under his directions until the Legislature could act upon his recommendation that the station be transferred to the Federal Government. This matter is now pending before the Legislature of that State, and successful action is expected on this recommendation before its adjournment. The shipping interests of this port would be greatly benefited immediately by the transfer of the quarantine to the Government, by the immediate cessation of all quarantine fees or tolls, now amounting to $2500 per month, also by having a medical inspection in effect from sundown to midnight, and further by having greatly-improved quarantine facilities and more prompt dispatch of vessels than heretofore. The foreign shipping interests of this port are greatly contributing, by their attitude and opposition to the transfer being effected now, toward the actual danger of the introduction of these dangerous contagious diseases.

Finally, as loyal citizens, interested in the welfare and protection of the health of our people, the foreign shipping interests owe to themselves the duty and obligation of co-operation in all beneficial measures, and should assist any proposed changes that will give better health protection to the city and the country.

[EDITOR'S NOTE.—Since the date of the above address the Legislature of New York has passed a bill authorizing the transfer of the New York Quarantine Station to the control of the United States Public Health Service, and subsequently, at the instigation of the Mayor, there was introduced in Council a measure to transfer to the same service the control of the Baltimore Quarantine.]

TONSILS AND ADENOIDS. Treatment and Cure. By Richard B. Faulkner, M.D., Columbia University. Pittsburgh, Pa.: The Blanchard Company. Paper. 1915.

This work is written from the standpoint of the physician and laryngologist in preference to that of the surgeon and laryngectomist. It is written by a physician of practical experience, and is published with the object of furnishing to careful physicians a medical line of treatment which has already secured positive curative results. It is a key to the work on "The Tonsils and the Voice." Though small, it is extremely practical, and should prove extremely useful to those needing help in gauging the proper medical treatment of diseased tonsils. Those who have already purchased "The Tonsils and the Voice" have the privilege of buying the above volume for one dollar.

INFANT WELFARE WORK: ITS NECESSITY —ITS REWARD.*

By *J. H. Mason Knox, Jr., M.D.,*

Associate in Clinical Pediatrics, the Johns Hopkins University.

THE activities of this week devoted to the welfare of the baby and young child, and which have been duplicated in many cities throughout the land, bring us additional proof, if such were needed, that the baby has at last "come to its own." This tiny unit in society, which from time immemorial has been the pride of its own mother and the recipient of much well-meaning advice from her mother and all the latter's friends, now takes its place as the most important potential member of society.

A Federal bureau has been organized in Washington to look after its interests, and many volunteer organizations devoted to various philanthropic and social projects are giving to the baby a large part, and in some cases all of their energies. We can start, then, with the thesis that it is of the utmost importance in this country of ours, if it is to survive and thrive in the future, to have many well babies born and to keep them well.

Though accurate statistics are notoriously lacking. it is thought that there is an infant population under one year of age in the United States of about 2,000,000 and an infant death rate for the same age period of about 150 per thousand, making a total of 300,000 infant deaths, nearly double the number who die from tuberculosis in all ages. The mere statement of these facts brings us at once face to face with the greatest health problem with which this country has to do. When we realize that the infant death rate in this country varies from 250 per thousand to less than 70, and throughout the world from between 400 and 500 per thousand in China to less than 40 in New Zealand, it is perfectly evident that the infant mortality rate is largely dependent upon conditions which can be controlled, at least in part, and that a large measure of responsibility attaches to any community whose baby death rate is unduly large. The death rate, in other words, is a *purchasable commodity.* It can be reduced to a minimum if the public is willing to pay the price. We must remember also that in the large majority of cases in which a forlorn and marantic baby is brought through its critical first year by proper care that the outlook for that baby is almost as good as that of any other: that its life expectancy is practically as long as that of a child who has been robust from birth, so that in the work of saving babies there is a greater incentive and a larger reward than is given to those engaged in other lines of preventive medicine. Without attempting

---

*Summary of address made during Child's Welfare Week, March 9, 1916. Medical and Chirurgical Faculty Building.

in any sense to be accurate, we can divide these 300,000 infant deaths into four large groups:

Those that die from—

(a)   Congenital debility, usually in the first weeks of life, about 75,000.

(b)   Gastro intestinal disorders, about 100,000.

(c)   Pulmonary disorders, about 75,000.

(d)   Various infections and other causes, about 50,000.

In Baltimore last year there were 16,355 infant deaths, the smallest number for many years.

Unquestionably, this national death rate could be cut in half if all the babies of the country were given even moderately efficient care. That is to say, that we are losing each year in the United States about 150,000 human lives at their very beginning because those who know, including national, State and municipal governments, and the better individual citizens, are not rendering effective aid to this dependent class of our population.

Let us discuss, briefly, some of the causes, general and specific, of this waste of baby life:

The two *general* causes everywhere recognized and always present when infant mortality rate is unduly high are: First—*Poverty*. This is a sad condition, and the solution of it should concern every thoughtful citizen. It presents difficulties which are far beyond the scope of this address. It can be said, however, that one of the strongest arguments in favor of the abolition of poverty, one of the greatest incentives in the effort to bring a fair competency within reach of every industrious family, is the crying need of the helpless babe. Repeated investigations have shown that the death rate under one year in families whose total earnings are less than $10 a week exceeds 250 per thousand, 1 to 4. Whereas, when the family income exceeds $25 a week, the infant death rate is but little over 80 per thousand, or about 1 to 13. ·

It is easy to imagine the effect of grinding poverty upon the health of a family. It means bad housing conditions, overcrowding, often immorality; it means the employment of mothers as wage-earners in factories or stores; it means the lowering of the standards of health, with increased nervousness and anxiety and an undercurrent of dread of the landlord, of grocery bill and of creditors in general, which creates an atmosphere in which it is very difficult to make a baby thrive. I am still old-fashioned enough to hope for an industrial regime throughout the country which will insure to the father or to him with the adult single members of the family a sufficient income to comfortably support the wife and younger children.

When this state of affairs arrives the infant in the family will have a better chance. Relief has been sought in many countries and in some of our own States through maternal insurance. The variety which seems best adapted to conditions in this country is a form of sick policy insurance, in which maternity, a period of several weeks before and after the baby's birth, is treated as illness.

In this way mothers are not obliged to work near the birth of their children.

The second general cause is *ignorance.* Nothing is more pitiable in visiting among the homes blessed by baby life than the widespread ignorance among young mothers concerning those matters that are essential to the baby's welfare. This, of course, is partly remedied by skilled attendance, but ignorance, together with poverty, make a combination very disastrous to the helpless baby. It fortunately is true that nearly all mothers, even though they may be ignorant, are interested and willing to learn. They always welcome the visit of a tactful physician or trained nurse. They are now learning inadequately and with difficulty after they have become mothers many things that they should have known in their school days.

If we would adequately reduce the infant death rate of the future, we must see to it that our older girls throughout the country are not permitted to leave school until they have received considerable instruction in personal hygiene and household economics, including the care of infants. When instruction of this kind is universal, much of this now necessary effort to instruct the mother in her home, often too late to save the baby, will become unnecessary.

There are, in addition, a number of specific causes leading to the loss of infant life, which can be briefly referred to.

First—*Diseased Parents.*—When we consider that a third of the total death rate in the first year occurs in the first month, and much of this among babies who are brought into the world too weak to live, because of inherited disease or weakness, it is high time to consider whether the public or the State should not take adequate means to prevent the marriage of the notoriously unfit. It is asking very little of the healthy to submit to a physical examination before marriage, when this general requirement means so much to the community. When we learn that more than one-fourth of all the premature babies born in a large obstetrical service are leutic, we have reached a time when the rights of the baby demand that we shall deal with this subject radically.

Second—*Overworked Mothers.*—It has been repeatedly shown that mothers who work immediately before confinement have smaller, less vigorous children, and that those who work immediately after confinement are much less able to care for their babies properly. It is the part of charity, nay rather of justice, to see that this abuse of nature's laws does not take place.

Third—*The Failure of Breast Milk.*—Here the physician is largely at fault. The difficulty of adjusting its mother's milk to the young infant, which is so often encountered in the first weeks of the baby's life, is made an excuse for weaning, in many cases unnecessarily. It has been found that 60 per cent. of working women in Baltimore, reached through our clinics, can nurse their babies for several months if encouraged and instructed to do so. It must be remembered that any bottle feeding substituted for breast milk requires a considerable degree of intelligence, an increased amount of time, money and more individual attention, all essentials which are difficult to obtain among the working people.

Fourth—*Impure Cow's Milk.*—Surely, if mother's milk fails, a self-respecting community should see to it that pure cow's milk is obtained for the new-born baby. It should be impossible for a mother to buy at public sale impure milk. Here she must be protected by carefully drawn and conscientiously enforced laws, because there may be nothing about the appearance of the milk to inform the purchaser that she is getting more of a poison than a food. Our milk supply in Baltimore has improved considerably in recent years, but it is still far short of a satisfactory product. It was the intention of those who were interested in having passed our present milk ordinance to give the Commissioner of Health sufficient power to enforce any milk standard he saw fit, and power to revoke any license on ten days' notice to a dealer or milk handler whose product fell below the required standard. In other words, it was the aim to concentrate in one person, the Commissioner of Health of Baltimore City, the responsibility for maintaining a satisfactory milk supply. It is most unfortunate that the legality of this ordinance has not been finally tested. In a number of instances, where the Health Commissioner has endeavored to exercise its powers as prescribed in the ordinance, he has been enjoined by the courts from proceeding further, and the wheels of justice move so slowly that no case has been finally tested in the Court of Appeals. It is very desirable that this should be done promptly, and if the ordinance is defective that another should be drawn, enlarging the powers of the Commissioner of Health. Baltimore is situated in the midst of an excellent dairy country, and could furnish its citizens better milk than any city of its size. Encouragement of breast nursing, and when this fails the use of properly modified cow's milk, up to the present time have been the most important factors in reducing infant mortality. The greatest reduction of infant death rate has occurred in the gastro-intestinal group. It is interesting to notice in Baltimore, from statistics recently compiled, that the very large increase in the number of infant deaths from gastro-intestinal disease taking place in the summer months has been greatly reduced in the last few years.

Fifth—*Crowded Dwellings.*—The close atmosphere which is found particularly in cold weather in so many homes, together with the overcrowding incident thereto, accounts for the great increase in deaths from pulmonary diseases among young infants in the winter. These deaths are almost as many in the winter as are those from gastro-intestinal disease in the summer. We are particularly negligent in the housing provisions offered to our colored population. This race, distinctly less resistant than the white, has double the white death rate and harbors all sorts of diseases, which are a continual menace, not only to themselves, but also to their white neighbors. Twenty-five per cent. of the colored babies born in Baltimore are born out of wedlock. The inadequate housing conditions, which the white race thrusts upon the negro, greatly encourage this immorality. Here, again, the claim of the baby should be heard voicing its protest against the exploitation of a weaker race.

Sixth—*Institutional Life.*—A word must be said concerning the care of very young babies, particularly the foundling and illegitimate child in institutions. Whenever this has been tried, even under fairly good conditions, the death rate has been enormous— 60, 70, 90 per cent. The truth is that the new-born baby requires individualizing care, which is very difficult, almost impossible to secure in a large institution. The practice which is so general in Maryland at present, of permitting the mother of an illegitimate child on the payment of a sum of money to place the child in an institution, sometimes before she has ever seen it, results usually in its speedy death, and in the waiving of maternal responsibility, which is hers, and which has been shown to be the most potent influence in helping her afterward to lead a normal life. The record of the Henry Watson Children's Aid Society, which has now cared for several hundred mothers and illegitimate children, with an infant death rate of about 5 per cent., is in marked contrast to the legalized slaughter which occurs in many large infant asylums.

Seventh—*Good Obstetrics.*—I have not referred to the baby's right to clean, skillful obstetrical care. From the lack of it hundreds of lives, of both mother and child, are unnecessarily lost. There is a crying need, which those much better equipped than I to discuss the subject have repeatedly emphasized, of thorough-going, radical reform in the handling of obstetrical cases among the working classes.

These are some of the important causes which at present needlessly destroy many infant lives. In the long future improved social conditions and, universal information concerning household economics and baby hygiene will result in the reduction of many of these ills, but there is much to be done in the present and in the immediate future. Today, in Baltimore, many babies are dying because their mothers do not know how or have not the means to keep them well. And it is just here that outside philanthropic organizations devoting themselves exclusively to the welfare of the baby are of the greatest help. This infant welfare movement was started 24 years ago in Paris, and has spread rapidly throughout all civilized countries. The main endeavor of them all is to bring advice and material help in the care of their babies to the mothers needing it.

Our Babies' Milk Fund Association in Baltimore was started by the Thomas Wilson Sanitarium in 1904. The first year's work was made possible by the generosity of Mr. Jacob Epstein. At first we had four stations and comparatively few babies. We have gradually grown to 16 stations, with as many nurses, and we reached in the course of last year over 7000 babies. Our nurses give their entire time to the care of infants and of children under three years of age. They have daily office hours in the stations, and respond to sick calls sent in by physicians and visit from house to house, instructing mothers how to feed and take care of 'their children.

In recent years, through co-operation with the large obstetrical clinics of the city, we have been able to come in contact with thousands of mothers before their babies were born. In these prenatal visits the nurse can see if adequate preparations have been made for the babies, whether the mothers have any abnormal symptoms requiring a physician's advice, and after the babies are born, as a friend, she can follow them with her advice and help throughout their infancy. Our welfare stations work in cordial co-operation with the city dispensaries and public clinics throughout the city. A nurse is assigned to the out-patient clinic of the Harriet Lane Home, and is prepared to help the mother in her own home carry out the dietary instructions given by the dispensary physician. Once or twice a week in each station consultations are held, in which mothers bring back their well babies for inspection and advice by physician and nurse.

In the summer months the Thomas Wilson Sanitarium is open to receive without charge any babies which are in need of hospital treatment in the country. These children are returned in convalescence to their homes under the direction of the nurses of the Babies' Milk Fund Association. During the last year, with the consent of the Health Commissioner of Baltimore City, the Babies' Milk Fund Association has had access to the birth registrations. By this means we are able to come in contact with many babies needing help which we either did not reach before, or perhaps only after they had become ill.

In Locust Point, a comparatively isolated district, an obstetrical clinic, under the charge of a well-trained physician, a woman, is being maintained, and her services are being much sought for.

In order to do this work adequately we should have almost twice as many nurses and stations. Does work such as is being done by the Babies' Milk Fund Association pay? In the last six years we have reached 26,137 babies, of whom 1300 have died. If the average city death rate had pertained among these babies 3300 would have died, so that one can see as the result of this single organization that approximately 2000 lives have been saved in six years. This work, let me repeat, must be looked upon as emergent in character. It *ought* not to be necessary, but until the wages of our working people are adequate to support their families in decency, until knowledge of baby care is made part of the mental equipment of every girl growing into maturity, work such as I have outlined is of more importance than that of any other department of preventive medicine, if we would save a constantly increasing number of babies to take their places among and share in the work of the succeeding generations of our citizens.

The Severn, Cathedral Street.

THE EFFECT OF VARIATIONS OF THE GASTRIC SECRETION UPON THE COMPOSITION OF THE SALIVA.

By Dr. T. R. Brown and Dr. E. B. Freeman.

WE both have been so interested in those peculiar affections of gums and tongue, gingivitis and glossitis, which are met with in a certain proportion of cases of achylia gastrica, and which play a considerable role in the symptomatology of pellagra and sprue, in which a gastric achylia is usually met with, that it seemed quite worth while to study the salivary secretion to determine whether there exists a relationship between the character of the gastric juice and the saliva.

The method we have employed has been the collection of all the saliva produced by the patient while chewing a piece of rubber of definite size, shape and weight for 20 minutes. This obviously is not especially physiological, and we may subsequently carry out a group of cases, using flavored gums, so that the sense of taste will play a role somewhat approximating that met with in the normal act of chewing.

In our experiments we determined the total amount of saliva, the degree of acidity or alkalinity and the amount of diastatic ferment contained therein, our idea being to find out, if possible, in the first place, whether we could establish a normal, and in the second place, whether permanent changes would be likely to be found in cases of long lasting hyperchlohydria, hypochlohydria and achylia.

Our series comprised 10 normal cases, 6 cases of subacidity, 10 cases of achylia gastrica, 6 of which showed either stomatitis or glossitis (only one of which was due to carcinoma of the stomach) and 15 cases of hyperchlorhydria.

In the *normal* cases the amount of secretion varied from 12 c.c. to 48 c.c., the average being 22.5 c.c.

The alkalinity of the saliva varied from 0 to 10, the average being 4, while in regard to the diastatic ferment, the last positive tube was the second in one case, third in two cases, fourth in two cases, fifth in one case and sixth in two cases.

Our method of determining the diastase was taking a 10 per cent. dilution of saliva in distilled water, and of this putting 2 c.c. in the first tube, 1 c.c. in the second tube, .7 c.c. in third, .4 c.c. in fourth, .2 c.c. in fifth, .1 c.c. in sixth, bringing up each tube to 2 c.c. with distilled water, adding 2 c.c. of 1 per cent. solution of soluble starch, incubating in the water bath at body temperature for one-half hour, then testing with a weak Lugol's solution.

The first negative tube is the first of the series in which the blue color shows that undigested starch is still present.

In the cases of *subacidity* the amount varied from 7 to 17 c.c., the average being 11.6 c.c.; the alkaline reaction from 0 to 16, the average being 6.3 c.c., while the last positive tube was No. 2 in one, No. 4 in two, No. 5 in one and No. 6 in three.

In the cases of *achylia* the quantity varied from 7 to 25 c.c., the average being 17.4 c.c.; the alkalinity from 2 to 10, the average being 6.8, while as to the diastase contents, the last positive tube was No. 2 in one case, No. 3 in two cases, No. 4 in two cases, No. 5 in four cases and No. 6 in one case (the last a case of carcinoma).

In the 15 cases of *hyperchlorhydria* the quantity varied from 7 to 55 c.c., the average being 20.4 c.c.; the alkaline reaction from 0 to 16, the average being 6.3, while as to the diastase, the last positive tube was No. 1 in one case, No. 2 in five cases, No. 4 in one case, No. 5 in one case and No. 6 in seven cases.

These figures show in the first place that the chewing of hard substances produces a considerable flow of saliva, quite rich in diastatic ferment, a view rather opposed to the general physiological opinion; second, that a consideration, as regards quantity, alkalinity and diastase contents in our cases of normal as compared to those of increased, diminished or absent hydrochloric acid in gastric contents, shows that in none of these are the variations from the normal sufficiently great to make us feel that there is any definite relationship between the character of the gastric juice and that of the saliva, and third, that it is not probable that qualitative, quantitative or ferment changes in the saliva play any considerable part in the development of glossitis, gingivitis and stomatitis, so frequently met with in cases of achylia gastrica.

We shall continue our investigation along two lines; first, carrying out similar studies after giving a substance which markedly stimulates the sense of taste; second, determining the pancreatic secretions in cases of achylia gastrica with and without lesions of the mucous membrane of the mouth to find out whether variations in the pancreatic secretions may play some part in the conditions.

CASES OF NORMAL GASTRIC SECRETION.

Cases.	Quantity.	Alkalinity.	Diastase.
1	12 c.c.	4	Tube No. 3 + No. 4 —
2	48 c.c.	0	Tube No. 4 + No. 5 —
3	25 c.c.	8	Tube No. 1 + No. 2 ± No. 3 —
4	10 c.c.	8	Tube No. 6 +
5	14 c.c.	0	Tube No. 5 + No. 6 —
6	21 c.c.	6	Tube No. 5 + No. 6 —
7	24 c.c.	2	Tube No. 3 + No. 4 ± No. 5 —
8	15 c.c.	2	Tube No. 5 + No. 6 +
9	45 c.c.	..	Tube No. 3 + No. 4 —
10	11 c.c.	10	Tube No. 4 + No. 5 —

CASES OF ACHYLIA GASTRICA.

1	14 c.c.	2	Tube No. 5 + No. 6 —
2	21 c.c.	4	Tube No. 5 + No. 6 —
3	20 c.c.	..	Tube No. 4 + No. 5 —

4	20 c.c.	8	Tube No. 3 + No. 4 —
5	7 c.c.	10	Tube No. 2 + No. 3 —
6	18 c.c.	..	Tube No. 5 + No. 6 —
7	20 c.c.	..	Tube No. 4 + No. 5 —
8	22 c.c.	..	Tube No. 3 + No. 4 —
9	25 c.c.	10	Tube No. 5 + No. 6 —
10	7 c.c.	..	Tube No. 6 +

CASES OF HYPOCHLOHYDRIA.

1	15 c.c.	16	Tube No. 2 + No. 3 —
2	17 c.c.	6	Tube No. 4 + No. 5 —
3	11 c.c.	4	Tube No. 5 + No. 6 —
4	9 c.c.	0	Tube No. 6 +
5	8 c.c.	6	Tube No. 4 + No. 5 —
6	14 c.c.	4	Tube No. 6 +
7	7 c.c.	8	Tube No. 6 +

CASES OF HYPERCHLORHYDRIA.

1	15 c.c.	8	Tube No. 2 + No. 3 —
2	18 c.c.	16	Tube No. 1 + No. 2 ± No. 3 —
3	18 c.c.	8	Tube No. 2 + No. 3 —
4	30 c.c.	8	Tube No. 6 +
5	20 c.c.	14	Tube No. 5 + No. 6 —
6	30 c.c.	4	Tube No. 6 +
7	17 c.c.	..	Tube No. 2 + No. 3 —
8	55 c.c.	..	Tube No. 1 + No. 2 —
9	22 c.c.	4	Tube No. 6 +
10	19 c.c.	0	Tube No. 6 +
11	7 c.c.	4	Tube No. 5 + No. 6 +
12	7 c.c.	4	Tube No. 3 + No. 4 ± No. 5 —
13	14 c.c.	2	Tube No. 6 +
14	20 c.c.	6	Tube No. 5 + No. 6 +
15	14 c.c.	4	Tube No. 2 + No. 3 —

Book Reviews.

POST-MORTEM EXAMINATIONS. By William S. Wadsworth, M.D., Coroner's Physician of Philadelphia. With 304 Original Illustrations. Philadelphia and London: W. B. Saunders Company. Baltimore: The Medical Standard Book Co. 1915. Cloth, $6 net. Half Morocco, $7.50 net.

Wadsworth's Post-Mortem Examinations enters into a thorough discussion of the technic and examination of the corpse. It deals with death and the changes in the dead body, and especially with the examination of the body from the first insertion of the post-mortem knife to the examination of the last organ, the skin, hair, head, brain, spinal cord, great vessels, organs of respiration, abdomen, etc. Besides it enters into a complete discussion of the medical legal aspects of post-mortems, such as the cause of death, coroner's examinations, medical evidence, abortion, asphyxia, burns and scalds, homicide, sexual crimes, etc. The entire art of making a scientific, systematic post-mortem is beautifully announced. As in other lines of medical endeavor, there is a right and wrong way of approaching the matter in hand. So in post-mortem examinations there is a right way to go about making the examination and getting the most information, and a wrong way. The author from an experience on more than 4000 bodies tells the right way, as well as the deductions to be drawn from the observations. It is a grand book, and should prove not only satisfactory to those doing post-mortems, but also from the attractiveness with which the subject is put, lead to a reawakening to the benefits to be derived from a careful exploration of the dead.

DISEASES OF THE SKIN. By Henry H. Hazen, A.B., M.D., Professor of Dermatology in the Medical Department of Georgetown University; Professor of Dermatology in the Medical Department of Howard University; Some Time Assistant in Dermatology in the Johns Hopkins University; Member of the American Dermatological Association. 233 Illustrations, including Four Color Plates. St. Louis: C. V. Mosby Company. 1915. Cloth, $4 net.

This book is somewhat over 500 pages, and contains a sufficiently fulsome account of the diagnosis, histo-pathology, etiology and treatment of those diseases of the skin which are met with in every-day practice. Its principal claim to recognition is the directness with which the author tackles his subject. Leaving out the wrinkles of the larger books and supplying more than the bare outline of the smaller ones, he hits a happy medium and supplies the reader with a sufficiency of the meat to allow of an intelligible understanding of the disease under discussion. It is well illustrated and extremely practical. With these perquisites it should easily worm its way into the affections of the student and general practitioner.

DIAGNOSTIC METHODS. By Herbert Thomas Brooks, A.B., M.D., Professor of Pathology, University of Tennessee, College of Medicine, Memphis, Tenn. Third Edition. Revised and Rewritten. St. Louis: C. V. Mosby Company. Cloth, $1 net. 1916.

As heretofore, this edition will be found a thoroughly reliable guide in diagnostic methods, namely, history taking, making of routine physical examinations and the usual laboratory tests necessary for students in clinical pathology, hospital interns and practicing physicians. It is no more or less than it pretends to be —a guide, giving merely the outlines and those methods found most useful in practical work. As such it will be found time-saving and very useful. To practicing physicians it affords a quick and reliable reference work on the subjects covered. For the price it cannot be duplicated.

MARYLAND MEDICAL JOURNAL

NATHAN WINSLOW. M.D.. *Editor.*

Associate Editors:

THOMAS R. BROWN. M.D.   JOSE L. HIRSH. M.D.
HUGH H. YOUNG. M.D.   A. SAMUELS. M.D.
RICHARD H. JOHNSTON. M.D.

BALTIMORE, JULY, 1916

CONGRATULATIONS.

BALTIMORE, the medical profession, and the Johns Hopkins University in special, are to be congratulated on the establishment by the Rockefeller Foundation of its school of hygiene and public health in connection with the Johns Hopkins University. The MARYLAND MEDICAL JOURNAL, on behalf of its readers and staff, rejoices in the fruition of this magnificent gift, a gift fraught with the utmost opportunities of assuaging the ills of mankind. As important as curative medicine is, its field is narrow to that of preventive medicine. It has taken many years of education to make the profession and the laity realize this, but the movement has within recent years been gaining ever and ever greater impetus, so that today it is generally accepted by the profession that more lives are to be spared and longevity prolonged by sanitary medicine—the opulence of riches and the meagerness of poverty, the betterment of the race, the problems of child labor, the restrictions on the exorbitant use of habit-forming drugs are soluble by sanitary medicine alone. Much has already been accomplished along these lines, but what has been done is insignificant to what is to be solved by concerted effort and investigation of the men who are now and will in the future devote their lives to this field of medicine. The opportunities placed in the hands of Dr. William H. Welch, the director of this new department, and his colaborers are inexhaustible. There is nothing of greater benefit to the human race than the curing of a sick man, but it is a thousand times more important to the community to prevent sickness rather than to cure it after it has developed. What can be done to prevent depletion of the race by preventive medicine has received an excellent object-lesson on a large scale on the Mexican frontier, where for a number of years a large body of men has been collected under the

(180)

auspices of the United States Army. Here typhoid, the scourge of the army in days gone by, is practically unknown. This has been brought about by proper sanitation and personal care bestowed on the men by the medical staff of the United States Army. The control and elimination of disease from the Isthmus of Panama, San Francisco, New Orleans, Cuba, etc., only evidences what sanitary medicine can accomplish. It is the hope of the inaugurators of the new department of the Johns Hopkins University that by study, collaboration and investigation the field of sanitary medicine will be still further broadened.

There is absolutely no means whereby the influence of this department for spreading the gospel of right living can be calculated. Every graduate and every person who is brought under its influence will be the center of an ever-widening circle of dissemination of the cult of natural living. Dr. Welch, in announcing the gift, said in part: "When we consider the revolutionary discoveries of the last forty years in our knowledge of the causes and means of prevention of diseases, the great progress in the science and art of public health and the incalculable benefits to the community in the application of this knowledge, we can all realize the beneficent service rendered to this great cause by the latest gift of the Rockefeller Foundation."

Inasmuch as the profession of the sanitarian and worker in public health, although closely connected, is not identical with that of the practitioner of medicine, the school of hygiene and public health, while working in co-operation with the medical school, as well as with the school of engineering, will have an independent existence under the university co-ordinate with these schools. The central and principal feature of the school will be an institute of hygiene housed in its own building, provided with the requisite laboratories and facilities, and with its own staff of teachers giving their entire time to the work of teaching and investigation. Occupational and industrial diseases, vital statistics, sanitary engineering, the diagnosis and handling of infectious diseases, infant mortality, child hygiene, mental hygiene, bacteriology, the chemical analysis of water and foods, energy analyses of foods, nutritional analyses of foods, environmental hygiene, climatological studies, etc., will be included in its scope. When one stops to meditate on the many activities to be served by the gift, then alone does one come to a thorough realization of the good to accrue to mankind through the generosity and foresight of the Foundation.

Medical Items.

DR. NATHANIEL M. KEITH, lately assistant to Dr. Hugh H. Young, director of the Brady Urological Clinic of Johns Hopkins Hospital, is in France with a section of the Harvard unit.

He left on May 20 and is supposed now to be on duty. He is the second Hopkins man to see service with the Harvard unit. Dr. Wm. D. Jack, the other, returned to Baltimore June 3 to take up work at the Brady clinic.

Dr. Keith was an intern at the clinic.

DR. LEE CHAPMAN BEAN, Johns Hopkins Medical School, '15, has been appointed assistant resident physician at the City Hospital, Bayview Asylum.

DR. FERDINAND O. W. REINHARD has returned to Baltimore after five months' Red Cross service in Serbia.

AT the fortieth annual commencement of the Johns Hopkins University at the Academy of Music, June 13, announcement was made by Dr. William H. Welch that the Rockefeller Foundation will establish its school of hygiene and public health in Baltimore in connection with the Johns Hopkins University. Dr. Wm. H. Welch will be the director of the school, with Dr. William H. Howell head of the physiological division. It is thought the school will open about October, 1917. It will be open to both men and women.

ANNOUNCEMENT has been made that Mr. Kenneth Dows of New York will give a large sum of money to Johns Hopkins University to establish and maintain a department for the study and prevention of tuberculosis. Of the amount given by Mr. Dows, $7500 is to be devoted to enlarging the laboratory facilities of the Phipps Tuberculosis Dispensary, which will be available at once. Then he has agreed to support the work of the dispensary by an annual contribution of $17,500.

Dr. Allen K. Krouse, Johns Hopkins Medical School, '07, who has had charge of the Trudeau Laboratory at Saranac Lake, N. Y., will come to Baltimore, and with a special staff will devote himself to this work.

DR HARRY M. SHIPLEY of Woodstock, Md., who has been confined to Mercy Hospital for a week suffering from kidney trouble, is some- what improved. An X-ray examination has been made, but it has not been decided whether an operation will be necessary or not.

DR. HOWARD A. KELLY has severed his connection with the Johns Hopkins Hospital for a year in order to devote all of his time to further research work in radium. Dr. Thomas S. Cullen will be in charge of Dr. Kelly's classes in the gynecologic department.

DR. MARTIN F. SLOAN, superintendent of the Eudowood Sanitarium, Towson, has opened offices in the Professional Building, Baltimore, for the practice of medicine. He will limit his practice to diseases of the chest.

DR. EUGENE W. HEYDE, Parkton, Md., has been appointed one of the health officers of Baltimore county to fill the vacancy caused by the death of Dr. Joseph S. Baldwin, Freeland, Maryland.

THE police commissioners of Baltimore city have elected the following physicians as surgeons to the board: Dr. Caleb N. Athey, president, and Drs. James M. Craighill, Wm. S. Gilroy, Thomas P. McCormick and Elliott H. Hutchins.

DR. BOWERS H. GROWT gave a reception to the members of the faculty and the members of the graduating class of the Medical School of the University of Maryland recently at his home.

THE Governor has reappointed Dr. Philip Briscoe, Mutual, Md., a member of the Board of State Aid and Charities.

THE first alumni and graduation banquet of the general alumni association of the University of Maryland was held May 31 at the Emerson Hotel and was attended by over 500 alumni and graduates. The following officers of the general alumni were elected for the ensuing year: President, E. John W. Revell; vice-president, Dr. Albert H. Carroll; treasurer, William K. Stichel; recording secretary, Dr. F. V. Rhodes; corresponding secretary, Edward P. Crummer, and advisory council, medical, Drs. Charles E. Sadtler, Arthur M. Shipley and James M. H. Rowland.

THE quarterly meeting of the Washington County Medical Society was held Thursday afternoon, May 11, at the Washington County

Hospital. Dr. E. Tracey Bishop of Smithsburg read a paper on "Proper Education in Regard to Medicine." Dr. J. Walter Layman of Hagerstown gave an account of the use of scopolamin in child birth in connection with the twilight sleep treatment. Dr. Hagg of New York read a paper.

THE engagement is announced of Paul Wilberforce Harrison, M.D., Johns Hopkins Medical School, of Bahrein, Arabia, to Miss Regina Rabbe, Union Protestant Infirmary Training School for Nurses, class of 1916. Dr. Harrison has been doing medical missionary work in Arabia for five years.

IF war is declared between this country and Mexico, Baltimore will likely lose many of its leading physicians, who will be called to the colors for service in the United States Medical Corps. Among them are:

Drs. Howard E. Ashbury, Charles F. Blake, John D. Blake, Charles J. Boehs, William A. Boyd, Samuel J. Fort, Edgar B. Friedenwald, John S. Fulton, Cary B. Gamble, Jr., Hubert C. Knapp, Edgar S. Linthicum, Duncan MacCalman, Standish McCleary, Alexius McGlannan, Firmadge K. Nichols, Isaac R. Pels, William W. Requardt, Arthur M. Shipley, Charles E. Simon, James E. Stowers, J. Harry Ullrich, Nathan Winslow, Randolph Winslow, Walter D. Wise, Harvey G. Beck, William S. Baer, Joseph C. Bloodgood, Thomas E. Chambers, Joseph A. Chatard, John M. T. Finney, William S. Halsted and William S. Thayer.

BIRTHS.

To WILLIAM T. CHIPMAN, M.D., University of Maryland Medical School, '12, and Mrs. Chipman of Felton, Del., May 22, 1916, a daughter—Mary Eloise.

To J. ALBERT CHATARD, M.D., Johns Hopkins Medical School, '03, and Mrs. Chatard, of 40 West Biddle street, May 27, 1916, a daughter—Octavia Whelan.

To HENRY J. WALTON, M.D., Baltimore Medical College, '06, and Mrs. Walton, of 720 West North avenue, June 9, 1916, a son—William Ellis.

MARRIAGES.

LLOYD WARREN KETRON, M.D., Johns Hopkins Medical School, '11, associate in dermatology, University of Maryland, of Baltimore,
Md., to Miss Romola Cressey of Modesto, Cal., at Baltimore, May 21, 1916.

ERNEST C. LEHNERT, M.D., University of Maryland Medical School, '02, to Miss Mabel Neily, both of Baltimore, Md., at Baltimore, June 7, 1916.

DEATHS.

JOHN EVELYN PAGE, M.D., University of Maryland Medical School, '89, surgeon (lieutenant commander), U. S. Navy (retired), of Santa Barbara, Cal., who entered the navy June 18, 1890, and was retired on account of incapacity resulting from an accident of service, April 3, 1903, after seven years and eleven months' sea service and six years and eight months' shore duty, died May 28, 1916, aged 49 years.

GEORGE HENRY CARPENTER, M.D., University of Maryland Medical School, '68, of Cumberland, Md., died in the Allegany Hospital of the Sisters of Charity, Cumberland, May 24, 1916, aged 73 years.

WILLIAM PAGE McINTOSH, M.D., surgeon, U. S. P. H. S., College of Physicians and Surgeons, '82, a Fellow of the American Medical Association and an active member of the Association of Military Surgeons of the United States, who entered the United States Public Health Service in November, 1885, was promoted to passed assistant surgeon, November 1, 1888, and to surgeon, May 20, 1890, and who was placed on waiting orders, April 15, 1915, on account of illness, died at Linwood, Howard county, Md., May 27, 1916, aged 60 years.

JOHN F. HANIFIN, M.D., College of Physicians and Surgeons, '11, of Holyoke, Mass., a member of the Massachusetts Medical Society, died in Saranac Lake, N. Y., May 7, 1916, from tuberculosis, aged 30 years.

DANIEL E. EVANS, M.D., Baltimore University, '92, of Nanticoke, Pa., formerly a member of the Medical Society of the State of Pennsylvania, died recently at his home, aged 66 years.

THOMAS S. GIBSON, M.D., University of Maryland Medical School, '87, of Alexandria, Va., died at his home, April 26, 1916, from cerebral hemorrhage, aged 56 years.

ANESTHESIA IN CHILDHOOD.

The Medical Council.

MANY authorities have taken occasion to direct attention to post-anesthetic vomiting. There have been numerous deaths reported from "delayed chloroform poisoning," and Nicloux and Fourquier have advanced an explanation resting upon the fact that chloroform is hydrolized by the alkalies of the blood, the reaction being as follows: $CHCl_3 + 3KOH = 3KCl + CO + 2H_2O$. In this reaction, as is readily seen, one molecule of chloroform combines with three of potassium hydrate in the blood, thus rapidly diminishing its normal alkalinity.

Vomiting is but one of the symptoms following chloroform narcosis, but an important one. In the case of children who vomit persistently following the administration of chloroform, one cannot get an alkali into the blood too soon, else fatty degeneration of the liver and death may follow.

It used to be thought that chloroform was the anesthetic of choice with children, but this view is losing ground. After one has had a couple frights during the administration of chloroform to children, as we have had, it is easy to become conservative in this regard. It is becoming just as important to learn *what happens to a drug* in the system as to find out what the drug does initially to the system, and the secondary action of drugs is an important study. This is especially true as regards narcotics and anesthetics.

Let us illustrate this. Perhaps some gentlemen thought we were severe in our arraignment of hydrated chloral in our June and July issues, but have they ever noted that in typhoid fever, *owing to the marked alkalinity of the tissues,* small doses of the drug are equal in effect to large ones in other diseases, and that in gout, owing to *the lack of alkali in the blood for its decomposition,* even large doses are not effective? We use this as an illustration because blood alkali is again involved, decomposing the drug into trichlor-ethyl alcohol. Also chloral hydrate causes degenerative changes in the liver, as does chloroform. The esters are subject to somewhat the same laws. Heroin is an acetic ester of morphin, and is incompatible with alkalies. It is subject to very erratic changes in the body, under certain conditions not well understood.

One could well get up quite an argument over the esters, such as ethyl nitrate, amyl nitrite, nitroglycerin, ethyl acetate, etc., all laying emphasis upon what happens to the drug in the system. Chloroform is $CHCl_3$ and methyl chlorid is CH_2Cl, produced by adding HCl to methyl alcohol, and it is an ester, as are others of the alcohols. Chloroform is made by heating ethyl alcohol with chlorid of lime; it is also made by distilling chloral with sodium hydroxid. Ether is also made from alcohol. In fact, the whole class of anesthetic drugs we have noted are related more or less with the alcohols, and what happens to them in the system is quite as important as is their ordinarily accepted physiological actions.

But to return to chloroform as administered to children, the line of study we have indicated is very vital, especially in this day of so much surgery in the diseases of children.

Argue as one may, chloroform is a dangerous anesthetic with

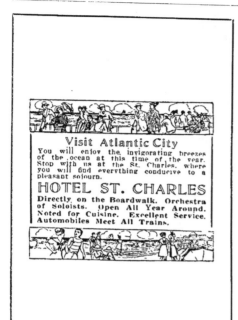
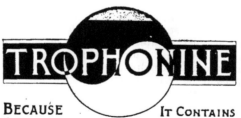

children. If it is used, never give rapidly, never use a mask, and never give in a sitting posture. Slow but continuous dropping upon gauze held several inches from the face is the best form of administration. Have oxygen and the tongue forceps handy.

Ether is decidedly safer than chloroform, except in bronchitis, heart and kidney lesions and tuberculosis. The open method with several layers of gauze has the disadvantage of chilling the ether vapor about 30° F., and in bronchitis the development of pneumonia is to be feared in consequence. The Cunningham apparatus, as described in the *Journal American Medical Association,* 1908, p. 1574, largely overcomes this difficulty. If the little patient be first purged and this apparatus used, very slight danger need be apprehended.

Tact and gentleness in administering ether to a child is important. Beginning gently with a little cologne, then a little ethyl chloride, and finally ether, will bring most children under with little or no struggle. But ethyl chloride must not be used to full anesthesia; it is too dangerous, the mortality being 1 to 1000. Ethyl bromide should never be considered, owing to its danger. Before removal from the operating table lavage may be practiced with advantage.

Nitrous oxide is ideal for short operations; it is safe, speedy, there is a lack of struggle and nausea and recovery from the effects is quick.

Dental surgeons are favoring nitrous oxide-oxygen anesthesia. While expensive for long operations, it does admirably. We have looked the matter up, tried to devise and secured the opinions of those with experience in the method; and it appears to be very safe and effective with children, although care must be exercised in case of a weak heart. It impresses operators as being safe in lung troubles, but not so effective as ether where muscular relaxation is a desideratum.

While commonly employed in adolescence, local anesthesia is not so well adapted to operations upon young children. The infantile tissues are readily devitalized, and freezing methods must be used with great care, if at all. Probably the application of ice and salt will produce a sufficient degree of cold for most cases in which freezing methods are applicable in children.. The sentiment of the profession seems to be more and more opposed to spinal anesthesia in children. Some authorities are using novocaine in infiltration anesthesia with children.

The special object of this article is to induce operators to refrain from such extensive use of chloroform in the practice of general anesthesia in children, and to prompt further study of what happens in the system to anesthetic and narcotic drugs. Our present knowledge along this line is very partial indeed.

THYMOL FROM HORSEMINT.

Government Specialists Find Commercial Possibilities in Development of New Industry.

THAT the commercial production in this country of thymol from horsemint may be, under favorable circumstances, a profitable undertaking is indicated by the recent investigations of the United States Department of Agriculture, the results of which are pub-

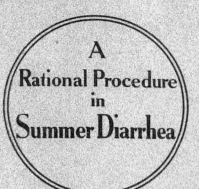
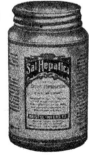

lished in Bulletin 372. Thymol is extensively used in medicine, and forms the basis of a number of important pharmaceutical compounds. In the past it has been imported from Northern Europe, where it is manufactured from ajowan seed grown in Northern India. Now that the European war has reduced these importations from over 18,000 pounds in 1914 to a little more than 2000 in 1915, it is believed that to some extent the demand can be supplied at home. For several years the Department of Agriculture has been conducting experiments with horsemint, which occurs as a common weed in many localities. These experiments have resulted in improving the plants by selection to a point which it is said warrants the use of horsemint for the commercial production of thymol.

Horsemint is found wild on light sandy soils over the entire region from Southern New York to Florida, and westward to Wisconsin, Kansas and Texas. It is probable that it will thrive under cultivation wherever it is found growing wild, but local economic conditions must be considered in determining whether or not its production would be profitable. The investigations of the Department of Agriculture indicate that by distilling the improved plants an average of 20 pounds of oil per acre may be obtained from first-year plantings, and that in succeeding years the yields should be at least 30 pounds per acre. The phenol content of this oil may be assumed to be about 70 per cent., almost all of which is thymol. The yields of thymol per acre of horsemint, therefore, should be for the first year a little less than 13 pounds, and for succeeding years a little less than 20 pounds. As the average price of thymol for a number of years has been about $2 a pound, the gross returns per acre from a horsemint plantation are estimated in the bulletin already mentioned at about $25.72 for the first year and $38.58 for each succeeding year.

It is more difficult to estimate with accuracy the cost of producing the thymol. In the opinion of the investigators, it is doubtful whether the profits from the industry will be sufficient to warrant anyone in engaging in it unless the horsemint is grown in connection with other oil-yielding plants for which a distilling apparatus is required. In that event, of course, the entire cost of the distilling plant cannot be charged against the thymol industry alone. For this reason in the estimates of cost of production published in Bulletin 372 such items as land rent, taxes, depreciation, upkeep and interest on the distilling plant have not been included. Excluding these items, it is believed that thymol can be produced at an approximate cost of $23 per acre the first year and $19 per acre thereafter. This figure includes the growing of the plants, fertilizer, cultivation, harvesting and distilling. A plantation of horsemint will not have to be replanted oftener than once in five years, and under average conditions may continue to give a good yield for a still longer time. After the first year a material reduction can be made in the cost of fertilizers if the distilled herb is returned to the soil. These facts account for the reduction in the cost of production after the first year.

Horsemint seed matures in the Southeastern States during August and September, and is ready to be gathered as soon as the calyx is dry and has assumed a dark brown color. The entire heads can readily be stripped off by hand. They should be spread out on a cloth or tight floor and thoroughly dried. The seed can then be removed by rubbing through a sieve, common window

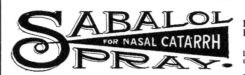

screening being about the right size. Where the winters are free
from severe frost and snow, as in the extreme Southeastern
States, the best results can be secured by planting the seed about
the first of September in a carefully-prepared seed bed. About
two months after sowing, when the plants are about two inches
high, they are ready for transplanting to the fields.

Fuller information in regard to methods of cultivation, harvesting and distilling are contained in Bulletin 372.

MEDICAL EDUCATION.

G. WILSON, Baltimore (*Journal A. M. A.,* April 8, 1916), after
noticing the raising of the standards within the past two decades
and admitting that the American people are receiving vastly better medical attention than even 10 years ago, says already the
cry for a doctor is coming from rural communities, and that they
are asking for a good doctor, if possible, but in any case a doctor.
While the report of the Carnegie Foundation on medical education in the United States has done an immense amount of good,
he thinks that it has held largely the position of an advocate
rather than of a judge, and has not considered sufficiently certain
important factors. One of these is the difference in the morbidity
rates in certain districts from those abroad and the bearing of the
per capita wealth of the community with the ratio of physicians
to population. His personal opinion as regards medical education
has been that there is need in this country of two classes of medical schools, the one like the Johns Hopkins, in which the requirements can hardly be set too high, and the other and larger class
for the training of general practitioners. The first type of school
should have a limited class of students, trained not only in clinical
and laboratory medicine, but also in the methods of research.
They would become teachers, research workers and specialists,
practitioners and consultants in the larger towns and cities. To
require this of all men who desire to practice medicine would,
Wilson thinks, undoubtedly raise the standard, but be no more
satisfactory than to require that all locomotive engineers be
graduates in mechanical engineering from an approved college.
The second class should demand a good education in the essentials, namely, the requirements demanded for admission to most
colleges and including the essential fundamental scientific branches
underlying medicine, such as chemistry, physics and biology. He
would not consider an ancient or modern language essential,
though it would be a help. He questions the general accuracy of
the statement of the Carnegie Foundation that graduates of the
Johns Hopkins Medical School have settled to any extent in small
communities. From a study of statistics he finds that they are
extremely rare in those of Maryland, where the other school in
Baltimore has 350 practitioners from its graduates. In 16 years,
from 1897 to 1913, inclusive, the Johns Hopkins Medical School
has graduated 965 men, of whom only four are practicing medicine in rural Maryland. He gives tables supporting the state-
ments, and trusts that the progress in regulating medical education will be done throughtfully, and quotes the words of President
Prichett of the Carnegie Foundation: "Let us not forget in our
zeal for research that the principal function of the medical school
is the training of medical practitioners." `

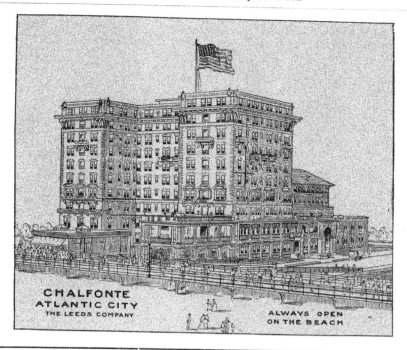
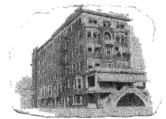

"HOW TO BLOW THE NOSE."

THERE is a lot of good sense in an article on blowing the nose contributed by Dr. E. Harrison Griffith to the *Medical Record*. There is no doubt that much trouble is caused to the nasal and accessory passages by the American habit of "hawking back" accumulated secretions into the nasopharynx. Back of the habit, however, is a very trying climate, and it is hardly likely the best-intentioned lecturers in the world will rid people of the almost uncontrollable impulse to get rid of irritant secretions in the easiest and apparently most natural way. We suggest that instead of lecturing us on the bad habits, the doctor should tell us what we may do to get rid of the unnatural condition that inspires it.

We confess that we feel a certain amusement at Dr. Griffith's suggestion that drills for the proper use of the handkerchief be instituted in the public schools. With toothbrush drills, handkerchief drills, breathing exercises and military maneuvers—and possibly other "drills" to come, and with hours set aside for religious instruction for lectures on sex hygiene, the poor youngsters will soon have no time to struggle with the "three R's." Juvenile human nature remains about the same from generation to generation, and the most powerful force in bringing up the child in the way he should go is the power of good example, which must begin at home. Don't try to crowd too much into the school course.

DO YOU KNOW THAT—

LIFE is a constant struggle against death?

Dirty refrigerators may make sickness?

The United States Public Health Service issues free bulletins on rural sanitation?

The defective citizen of today is ofttimes the unhealthy child of yesterday?

Every man is the architect of his own health?

It's the baby that lives that counts?

Tuberculosis is contagious, preventable, curable?

The full dinner pail—the open window—the clean well—make for health?

Light promotes cleanliness?

A clean mouth is essential to good health?

Physical training in childhood is the foundation of adult health?

The U. S. Public Health Service issues publications on hygiene and sanitation for free distribution?

Isolation is the most efficient means of controlling leprosy?

Headache is Nature's warning that the human machine is running badly?

Bullets may kill thousands—flies tens of thousands?

Obesity menaces longevity?

Walking is the best exercise—and the cheapest?

The United States Public Health Service administers typhoid vaccine gratis to Federal employees?

A little cough is frequently the warning signal of tuberculosis?

Bad teeth and bad tonsils may be the cause of rheumatism?

Unpasteurized milk frequently spreads disease?

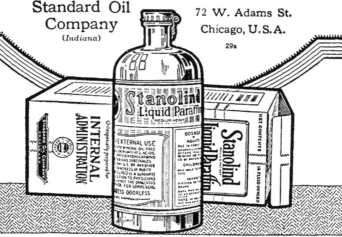

Publishers' Department.

Danger Due to Substitution.

HARDLY another of all the preparations in existence offers a wider scope to imposition under the plea of "just as good" than the scientifically standardized Eucalyptol.

The most recent fraud practiced in regard to this product is an attempt to profit by the renown of the firm of Sander & Sons. In order to foist upon the unwary a crude oil, that had proved injurious upon application, the firm name of Sander & Sons is illicitly appropriated, the make-up of their goods imitated, and finally the medical reports commenting on the merits of their excellent preparation are made use of to give the desired luster to the intended deceit.

This fraud, which was exposed at an action tried before the Supreme Court of Victoria at Melbourne, and others reported before in the medical literature, show that every physician should see that his patient gets exactly what he prescribed. No "just as good" allowed.

In Functional Nervous Diseases.

THE first and fundamental question which the earnest physician asks today in determining the utility of any remedy he wishes to use is "what will it accomplish?" If it does what he asks it to do, and does it better than anything else he has ever employed, he will certainly use it in preference to anything else. If it fails and proves valueless, he will as certainly discard it in short order. His common sense and intelligence will permit of no other course, for medical men build their practices on successes, not on failures. Beneficial results of a definite, positive character are constantly sought, and it is in achieving these that a physician proves his worth as a practitioner of medicine. Thus in the treatment of functional nervous diseases derangement of the bodily nutrition is so prominent a factor that the first consideration in these affections is a restoration of the nutritional balance. To accomplish this Gray's Glycerine Tonic Comp. is widely recognized as a remedy of remarkable efficiency. Under its systematic use the appetite is increased, the digestion is improved and the nutrition shows a marked and substantial gain. Coincident with this nutritional gain there is a corresponding increase in nerve force, with a very pronounced and grati-

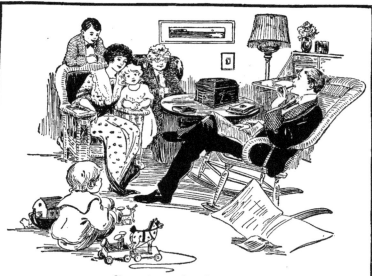

fying correction of insomnia, indigestion, head-
aches, vague pains, nervousness and other
symptoms of nervous origin.

If you have some case of neurasthenia or
other functional nervous disease and would like
to give Gray's Glycerine Tonic a critical trial,
why not send today for samples? A supply will
be sent you at once. Address the Purdue Frederick Co., 135 Christopher St., New York.

Campetrodin.

THIS preparation is an oleaginous solution of
iodine in camphor. Soothing, penetrating, powerful antiseptic, local analgesic, alterative, ideal
surgical dressing.

The great therapeutic value of Campetrodin
is attributed to the fortunate properties of its
vehicle, which permits the remedy to enter the
tissues and blood stream, as it were, by osmosis,
bringing about results immediate and satisfactory. Wherever the therapeutic properties of
iodine are indicated, Campetrodin can be relied
upon, minus the disadvantage of crude iodine.
It relieves local pain promptly without local
irritation; on the contrary, it can be applied to
denuded or burned surfaces as an anodyne.
As an antiseptic dressing it is equal to any,
and without the dangers of most of them. In
all cases where prompt absorption or lymphatic
stimulation is desired it penetrates the tissues
almost as soon as it is applied to the skin.

Campetrodin (Double Strength) is especially
valuable in reducing swollen glands and relieving obstinate, deep-seated rheumatic and
neuralgic pains.

Both strengths supplied on prescription in
one, three and eight ounce bottles.

On request the manufacturers, A. H. Robins
Company, Richmond, Va., will be glad to send
samples for clinical test.

A Notable Germicide.

IT is becoming more and more apparent as
time passes that in Silvol we have a germicide
of uncommon usefulness. Its field embraces
practically all inflammations of mucous mem-
branes. The indications for Silvol include con-
junctivitis, corneal ulcer, trachoma, rhinitis,
sinus infections, otitis media, pharyngitis, ton-
sillitis, laryngitis, gonorrhea, cystitis, posterior
urethritis, vaginitis, cervical erosions, endome-
tritis, etc.—all infections, in short, in which a
silver salt is applicable.

Silvol would appear to have a number of advantages over most of the other proteid-silver compounds. It is freely soluble in water. While an exceptionally powerful antiseptic, it is non-irritating in ordinary dilutions. Silvol solutions are not precipitated by proteids or alkalis or any of the reagents that commonly affect other silver compounds in solution. They do not coagulate albumin or precipitate the chlorides when applied to living tissue.

In the treatment of acute inflammations of mucous membrane Silvol may be used locally in solutions as strong as 50 per cent. with very little pain or irritation. In inflammatory affections of the ear, nose and throat it may be used in 5-to-40-per-cent. solution, and for irrigating sinuses a 2-to-5-per-cent. solution may be employed with benefit. For inflammatory conditions of the eye and conjunctival infection with pneumococci and staphylococci a 10-to-40-per-cent. solution may be applied with benefit three times a day. In acute gonorrhea, as an abortive measure, a 20-per-cent. solution should be injected every three hours, while in the routine treatment the injection of a 5-per-cent. solution three times a day is recommended.

Silvol is a Parke, Davis & Co. product. It is supplied in ounce bottles and in bottles of 50 capsules, each capsule containing 6 grains; also in ointment form (5-per-cent. Silvol) in collapsible tubes containing approximately ⅛ ounce and 1¼ ounces.

Codliver Oil for Children.

OWING to its very acceptable character, Cord. Ext. Ol. Morrhuæ Comp. (Hagee) is especially adapted for use as a reconstructive in children. Either as a tissue-maker in debilitated conditions resulting from impaired metabolism or consequent upon an acute illness, Cord. Ext. Ol. Morrhuæ Comp. (Hagee) will prove of marked advantage. Its therapeutic powers are added to by its palatability. It may be continued over long periods without causing gastric distress, nor does the hot weather make its use more difficult.

More Than a Coincidence.

IT was more than a coincidence that thousands of physicians stated in response to a recent inquiry that one of their most highly-prized drugs was cactus. A few doctors might have so reported and the fact be attributed to personal prejudice, but when the same is vouch-

safed by thousands of earnest practitioners, it must be believed that their verdict was based on actual observation and clinical experience.

There can be no doubt that Cactina Pillets fill a definite place in the management of cardiac disorders. No claim is made that these are to supersede the more powerful cardiac drugs, when these are properly indicated, but when it is desired to support and sustain the heart and strengthen and regulate its action, Cactina Pillets will not disappoint. Thus a great many physicians have grown to look on Cactina Pillets as one of the safest and most satisfactory cardiac tonics at their command. One to two Cactina Pillets every three or four hours will be found excellent—for example, for relieving the so-called "tobacco heart."

Fretful Children.

WHILE in the majority of instances fretfulness in children points to the need of correcting—for instance, some gastro-intestinal disorder—yet there are times when a sedative is indicated, and at such times the physician will find PASADYNE (Daniel) of more than ordinary value. PASADYNE (Daniel) is merely a distinctive name for a pure, concentrated tincture of passiflora incarnata. While therapeutically active, PASADYNE is free from danger, a point that gives it a particular advantage in children.

Following its administration, these little patients secure restful sleep.

A sample bottle may be obtained by addressing the laboratory of John B. Daniel, Inc., Atlanta, Georgia.

Iodine in Syphilis.

WHILE the extraordinary worth of iodine in late syphilis easily places it among the indispensable therapeutic agents made use of by modern medicine, yet it is due to the skill of the pharmaceutical chemist that iodine has been enabled to hold its high rank as a drug agent. Iodine as such, of course, is out of the question, and even the popular iodide of potash oftentimes occasions such distress as to neutralize its potential value. But in IODIA (Battle) the physician has an iodine product of distinct usefulness, and particularly in the later manifestations of syphilis, for not only does it provide a means of introducing iodine into the system, but, furthermore, it is free from the irritating qualities of the plain iodide. Its therapeutic effects are further enhanced by the addition of certain of the vegetable alteratives which have been clinically shown to exert an influence on the syphilitic processes. Whenever iodine is indicated, IODIA (Battle) may be exhibited with decided benefit.

A Systemic Boost.

IT is safe to say that the average physician is called upon to prescribe a tonic more frequently than any one other form of medication, unless it be a cathartic. Patients who are patients solely because they are tired, "run down" and generally debilitated are constant visitors at the physician's office. Such individuals need something that will boost them up to their normal point of resistance and then hold them there; in other words, not a mere temporary stimulation, with secondary depression, but a permanent help to the revitalization of the blood and a general reconstruction. Pepto-Mangan (Gude) is not only prompt in action as an encourager of appetite and better spirits, but is also distinctly efficient as a blood builder and systemic reconstituent. It is pleasant, non-irritant, free from constipating effect and does not stain the teeth. It is thus a general constitutional tonic of positive service in all conditions of general devitalization.

Sleeplessness.

THERE can be no denying the fact that for all-round use, the bromides still hold first place in the rational treatment of insomnia. Of course, especial care should be used in selecting the particular bromides to be employed, as the results accomplished obviously depend to a large extent on their purity and quality. This is well shown by the notable therapeutic utility of Peacock's Bromides, a preparation of bromide salts that for many years has been the first remedy turned to by countless discriminating physicians whenever a sedative or hypnotic has been needed. Particularly in overcoming the sleeplessness due to nervous excitation, neurasthenia, alcoholism, prolonged worry, hysteria, and so on, have Peacock's Bromides been found of never-failing efficiency, with gratifying freedom from gastric irritation, and the all too evident drawbacks that so often characterize other hypnotic agents.

Mellin's Food

was the first preparation of maltose and dextrins presented to physicians in serviceable form, and it stands today as a true representation of Liebig's principles, which are now so generally applied to scientific infant feeding.

"I HAVE used Tongaline for more than 20 years and have found it most satisfactory in every way. A very recent case which came under my care was one in which several physicians had failed, even with the use of organotherapy. Within 48 hours after Tongaline had been administered there was a decided remission of temperature and pain and at the end of one month the patient, who was a lady about 70 years of age and had been a sufferer for years, was able to go about her room and to comb her own hair—something which she had not done for six months previously."

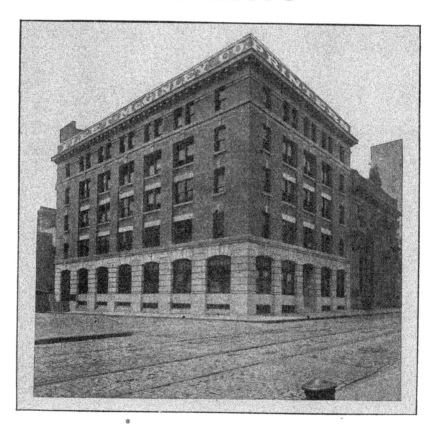

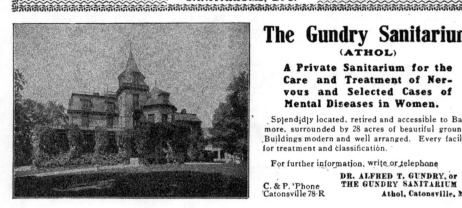

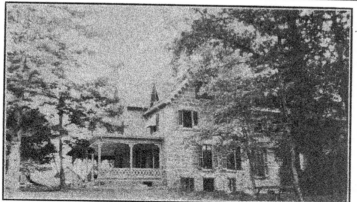
¶ When you write advertisers, mention the MARYLAND MEDICAL JOURNAL.

University of Maryland School of Medicine and College of Physicians and Surgeons

Faculty of Physic

RANDOLPH WINSLOW, A.M., M.D., LL.D., Professor of Surgery.

L. E. NEALE, M.D., LL.D., Professor of Obstetrics.

CHAS. W. MITCHELL, A.M., M.D., Professor of Pediatrics and Clinical Medicine.

THOS. A. ASHBY, M.D., LL. D., Professor of Diseases of Women.

JOHN HOLMES SMITH, M.D., Professor of Anatomy.

JOHN C. HEMMETER, M.D., Ph.D., Sc.D., LL.D., Professor of Physiology and Clinical Medicine.

A. M. SHIPLEY, M.D., Professor of Materia Medica and Surgical Pathology.

S. K. MERRICK, M.D., Professor of Diseases of the Nose and Throat.

R. B. WARFIELD, M.D., Professor of Practice of Surgery.

GORDON WILSON, M.D., Professor of Principles of Medicine.

WILLIAM SIMON, Ph.D., M.D., Sc.D., Professor of Chemistry.

JOHN W. CHAMBERS, M.D., Sc.D., Professor of Surgery.

NATHANIEL G. KEIRLE, A.M., M.D., Sc.D., LL.D., Professor of Medical Jurisprudence.

WILLIAM F. LOCKWOOD, M.D., Professor of Medicine.

GEORGE W. DOBBIN, A.B., M.D., Professor of Obstetrics and Gynecology.

WILLIAM ROYAL STOKES, M.D., Sc.D., Professor of Pathology and Bacteriology.

HARRY FRIEDENWALD, A.B., M.D., Professor of Ophthalmology and Otology.

ARCHIBALD C. HARRISON, M.D., Professor of Surgery.

CARY B. GAMBLE, JR., A.M., M.D., Professor of Clinical Medicine.

WILLIAM S. GARDNER, M.D., Professor of Gynecology.

STANDISH McCLEARY, M.D., Professor of Pathology.

JULIUS FRIEDENWALD, A.M., M.D., Professor of Gastroenterology.

J. M. H. ROWLAND, M.D., Professor of Clinical Obstetrics.

ERNEST ZUEBLIN, M.D., Professor of Experimental and Clinical Medicine.

JOSE L. HIRSH, B.A., M.D., Professor of Clinical Pediatrics.

HIRAM WOODS, JR., M.A., M.D., Professor of Eye and Ear Diseases.

JOHN S. FULTON, A.B., M.D., Professor of State Medicine.

HARRY ADLER, B.A., M.D., Professor of Clinical Medicine.

THOMAS C. GILCHRIST, M.R.C.S., M.D., Professor of Dermatology.

FRANK MARTIN, B.S., M.D., Professor of Operative and Clinical Surgery.

CHARLES G. HILL, A.M., M.D., Professor of Psychiatry.

A. C. POLE, M.D., Professor of Descriptive Anatomy.

J. D. BLAKE, M.D., Professor of Clinical Surgery.

J. FRANK CROUCH, M.D., Professor of Clinical Ophthalmology and Otology.

CHARLES O'DONOVAN, A.M., M.D., LL.D., Professor of Clinical Pediatrics and Clinical Medicine.

G. MILTON LINTHICUM, A.M., M.D., Professor of Proctology.

W. B. PERRY, M.D., Professor of Clinical Gynecology.

TILGHMAN B. MARDEN, A.B., M.D., Professor of Histology and Embryology.

J. MASON HUNDLEY, M.D., Professor of Clinical Gynecology.

JOSEPH T. SMITH. M.D., Professor of Hygiene.

R. TUNSTALL TAYLOR, M.D., Professor of Orthopedic Surgery.

JOHN R. WINSLOW, B.A., M.D., Professor of Diseases of the Throat and Nose.

J. M. CRAIGHILL, M.D., Professor of Clinical Medicine.

JOS. E. GICHNER, M.D., Professor of Clinical Medicine and Physical Therapeutics.

CHAS. M. McELFRESH, M.D., Professor of Clinical Medicine.

IRVING J. SPEAR, M.D., Professor of Nervous Diseases.

JAMES A. NYDEGGER, M.A., M.D., ScD., Surgeon U. S. P. H. Service, Professor of Tropical Medicine.

GIDEON TIMBERLAKE, M.D., Professor of Genito-Urinary Diseases.

EDWARD N. BRUSH, M.D., Professor of Psychiatry.

C. HAMPSON JONES, M.B., C.M. (Edinburgh), M.D., Professor of Hygiene and Public Health.

JOHN RUHRAH. M.D., Professor of Pediatrics.

CHARLES F. BLAKE, A.M., M.D., Professor of Proctology.

CHARLES E. SIMON, A.B., M.D., Professor of Clinical Pathology and Experimental Medicine.

FRANK DYER SANGER, M.D., Professor of Diseases of the Throat and Nose.

BARTGIS McGLONE, A.B., Ph.D., Professor of Physiology.

G. CARROLL LOCKARD, M.D., Professor of Clinical Medicine and Director of Medical Clinic.

SAMUEL J. FORT, M.D., Professor of Materia Medica and Pharmacology.

JOHN G. JAY, M.D., Clinical Professor of Surgery.

NATHAN WINSLOW, A.M., M.D., Clinical Professor of Surgery.

PAGE EDMUNDS, M.D., Clinical Professor of Genito-Urinary Diseases.

WILLIAM TARUN, M.D., Clinical Professor of Ophthalmology and Otology.

CHARLES E. BRACK, Ph.G., M.D., Clinical Professor of Obstetrics.

HARVEY G. BECK, Ph.G., M.D., Clinical Professor of Medicine.

ALBERTUS COTTON, A.M., M.D., Clinical Professor of Orthopedic Surgery and Roentgenology.

ALEXIUS McGLANNAN, A.M., M.D., Clinical Professor of Surgery and Surgical Pathology.

ANDREW C. GILLIS, A.M., M.D., Clinical Professor of Neurology and Psychiatry.

For further information, apply to **WM. F. LOCKWOOD, M.D.**, Dean of the Faculty, or **CALEB WINSLOW, M.A.**, Registrar. University of Maryland School of Medicine and College of Physicians and Surgeons, Baltimore, Md.

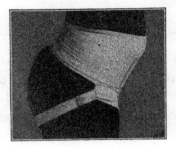

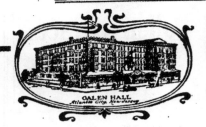

CPSIA information can be obtained
at www.ICGtesting.com
Printed in the USA
BVHW04*1047170918
527708BV00015B/1964/P